NEW CHOICES, NEW CHANCES

NEW CHOICES, NEW CHANCES

REVISED EDITION

A Woman's Guide to Conquering Cancer

RITA ESPOSITO WATSON
and
ROBERT C. WALLACH, M.D.

St. Martin's Press *New York*

For chapter review of updated material, my thanks to Jennifer Kelsey, Ph.D.; Nancy Hildreth of Yale's Department of Epidemiology and Public Health; Jay Katz, M.D., of the Yale Law School; also Beatrice LoFrita-Heyde; and our editor Karen Johnsen. A special thanks to all the women who graciously shared their stories with us—for you.

—REW

Design by Ed Kaplin

Library of Congress Cataloging in Publication Data

Watson, Rita Esposito.
New choices, new chances.

1. Generative organs, Female—Cancer. 2. Generative organs, Female—Cancer—Prevention. 3. Women—Health and hygiene. I. Wallach, Robert C. II. Title.
RC280.G5W37 616.99'465 81-16746
ISBN 0-312-56604-2 (pbk.) AACR2
ISBN 0-312-56603-4

Revised Edition
10 9 8 7 6 5 4 3 2

This book is dedicated to our sons—
and the women in their lives—may they
all benefit from knowledge and progress
in the fight against cancer.

RCW REW

Contents

Introduction

Women's outlook on health, childbirth, and sexuality has changed dramatically in the last ten to fifteen years. We have come to see that we have a right to know about our own bodies and health.

It seemed simple enough for us to learn about the normal female functions from menarche to menopause. Yet our medical education seemed to stop short when it came to learning about cancer. Cancer was too complex or too frightening even to discuss. For too long cancer was dreaded as an inevitably fatal disease. Many women would just say, "If you're going to get it, you're going to get it. Why worry about it before it happens?"

Today, however, more and more women are learning that the better informed one is about cancer:

- the less likely it is that you will worry needlessly about it;
- the more likely you will be to recognize for which cancer, if any, you may be at a higher risk;
- the more likely you will be to take the preventive measures necessary to keep yourself cancer-free;
- the better able you will be to trust yourself and your decision-making ability should you, one day, be diagnosed as having cancer.

The more a woman knows about herself and her health, the better able she is to work with her physicians, and with the doctor within her—that inner voice, call it, if you like, intuition—when she is faced with decisions about medical treatment.

I would like to be able to say that since we wrote this book, treatment procedures have undergone a revolutionary change. Unfortunately they have not. One year after the hardcover edition of this book first appeared, there is still no infallible cure for cancers of the breast and reproductive system. Less radical treatments for breast cancer are being given serious consideration, but the issue is still under debate.

New studies do appear all the time, and although none of them alter the content of this book, some of them will no doubt be of interest to women who want to learn more about specific topics. We have included listings of some of the most important studies—those most accessible to the lay reader—at the end of the individual chapters on cervix, breast, and estrogen cancer.

While no treatment breakthroughs have as yet materialized, there has been a thoughtful and critical evaluation of the role of informed consent. Throughout this book we talk about the need to be informed—to work within a patient/doctor partnership. Now, in a report called *Making Health Care Decisions* from a Congressionally-mandated commission,* the issue of informed consent and patient-doctor partnerships has been brought into proper perspective in what is called "shared decision-making." Before you can participate in the decision-making process, however, you must have accurate and adequate information concerning the disease, treatment options, and alternatives.

Through my own work with women, and through reporting on health issues, I have come to see that the women—and also the men—who were able to conquer cancer had a formula for success. These individuals were:

- determined to become victors not victims

***Making Health Care Decisions: The Ethical and Legal Implications of Informed Consent in the Patient-Practitioner Relationship*, a report from The President's Commission for the Study of Ethical Problems in Medicine and Biomedical and Behavioral Research.

• aggressive enough to find competent physicians with whom they could work

• willing to learn everything they could about the disease and available treatments

• able to maintain a positive attitude.

Finding a competent physician is a crucial task. Developing a relationship with that physician (or physicians) may be one of the greatest challenges. Often when cancer is diagnosed, you are sent to a specialist who has little time to spend learning who you are as a woman. The specialist will rarely be the family doctor who knows you well enough to know whether you want to be told every detail—or no details. The woman with a newly diagnosed cancer owes it to herself to be straightforward and assertive with the physician.

Clarification of my own thinking on the issue of informed consent came as the result of a class at the Yale Law School. I have come to see that my view of the competent physician was somewhat naive. When we wrote about choosing a physician in Chapter Two we perhaps assumed that the competent physician would of course be a communicating physician. This is not necessarily the case.

What we stress throughout this book—getting accurate and adequate information—is taken a step further by the Ethics Commission. You not only have the right to know, you have the right to take part in decision-making. The issue is not merely one of disclosure—that is, being told all that you need to know—it is one of consent as well. To most of us "consent" means signing a form written in some mysterious medicalegalese jargon giving the physician permission to treat you. Consent should take on a new meaning, one that says, "I understand and I agree."

Sometimes women feel that their physicians are such busy people that they shouldn't trouble them to explain terms and procedures that they do not understand. Some women feel that asking too many questions will just make the doctor angry. Remember, it is every woman's right to know about any disease that affects her body. It is your right to know how your physician proposes to treat those diseases and what alternatives exist if you decide against treatment.

The Commission noted that "the ethical foundation of informed consent can be traced to the promotion of two values: personal well-being and self-determination. To ensure these values are respected and enhanced, the Commission finds that patients who have the capacity to make decisions about their health care must be permitted to do so voluntarily and must have all relevant information regarding their condition and alternative treatments, including possible benefits, risks, costs and other consequences, and significant uncertainties surrounding any of this information."

So it is really up to you. It is your responsibility to inform yourself of some basic health facts and then ask yourself:

- Do you want to be involved in a patient-doctor partnership?
- Do you want your physician to tell you everything there is to know about treatments and treatment options?
- Do you want to know what side effects might accompany each treatment?
- Do you want to know the alternatives?
- Do you want to know the risks as well as the benefits?

You should want to know. And since in some instances a physician can be legally justified in giving "less than full disclosure," you should make your physician aware of your desire to be told. Why should you want to be told anything or everything? Some treatments are irreversible. You cannot, for instance, decide you want breast cancer treated by radiation only, after you've consented to and had a mastectomy. You cannot decide you want to conceive a child after a hysterectomy. But you can decide you want a hysterectomy after trying less radical treatment—conization—for cervical cancer.

To facilitate the shared decision-making process, we present in this book questions to ask and answers to expect. We try not to let our own preferences for a particular type of treatment or no treatment influence you. It is your body.

What about a physician's preferences towards a particular treatment? Should you let his or her opinion influence you? Maybe yes, if you are truly undecided. If you have a competent physician whom you trust and you are not opposed to his or her treatment choices, there is, perhaps, no need to seek out other physicians. In an ideal relationship, the physician will be sensitive to your needs, respect your wishes, and assist you in the decision-making process.

This book, then, should be used as a source book, a guide to help you talk to your doctor. It is meant to give you a basis for a meaningful dialogue. In reading this book we suggest you determine:

- For what type of cancer might I be at risk?
- How might I reduce that risk?
- Do I have a primary care physician whom I can trust to refer me to a cancer specialist?
- If I am told that I have cancer, what choices are available to me?

Should you be diagnosed as having cancer, work with your physician sufficiently so that you understand what treatments you are consenting to. Understand the consent forms. The Commission suggests you and your physician might want to draft a consent form prior to hospitalization. This gives you the opportunity to read a document in clear, nontechnical language.

Be aware that the type of treatments you receive may dramatically affect your quality of life. Adequate information on the various treatments and their side-effects is within every woman's reach. Only with such information can a woman make an informed choice, one that will give her a certain peace of mind.

I look to women to turn the tide against cancer in this country. I think it can happen. I think it is happening. Am I taking an overly feminist attitude? I thought so until I found that the male physician who delivered my children agreed with my theory. It was he who taught me to question and to expect answers regarding my pregnancies. It was he who taught me to see the importance of women learning about their bodies. He is a gynecologic oncologist, and it was with him that I discovered that women asking the right questions and expecting answers can help to conquer cancer. Together we wrote this book.

Rita Esposito Watson

Chapter One

What Is Cancer?

Jane's victory over cancer is the type of success story that everyone likes to read about. Ten years ago she was told that she had only a few months to live. For a nineteen-year-old full of dreams, the news was nightmarish.

On her eighteenth birthday Jane had married and with her husband, director of a well-established import-export company, moved to America from France. Although she wanted to begin her family immediately, it took Jane about a year to conceive. Before announcing the happy news that she was expecting, she went to see an obstetrician recommended by an associate of her husband's. The physician also happened to be a specialist in female cancer.

Jane was examined, and the physician realized that her uterus was too large for a woman who claimed to be only three months pregnant. He suspected and later correctly diagnosed a rare malignant tumor called choriocarcinoma, which in many ways mimics pregnancy. While it is rare in the United States, choriocarcinoma has been a major health problem in other parts of the world. At the time of her diagnosis, Jane's malady was often considered fatal. The physician suggested immediate treatment with drugs that today are recognized as "the cure" for this rare tumor.

Jane never gave up hope. Despite some time in the hospital and the unpleasant side effects of the drug, she kept up a very positive attitude. Today, at twenty-nine, Jane has just given birth to her third healthy child. Cancer has not interfered with her marriage, parenting, nursery school activities, work for a women's organization, and Sunday-school teaching schedule.

The happy outcome of Jane's story is not unusual. For women with many kinds of cancer, rare as well as common; there is more than just hope. There is the probability of cure. Today, more women than ever before are conquering cancer. Each day newspapers carry stories of new drugs, new treatments, new techniques, and new means of identifying cancer-causing agents. All this is helping women with cancer to live longer and to enjoy healthier lives.

While we are always happier to read the success stories of women like Jane, this book came to be written because of the three women mentioned in the introduction. Their stories are very different.

Susan was a bright, well-educated wife and mother. She developed a series of symptoms that appeared to indicate the presence of cancer. Her physician recommended a biopsy, the removal of a small section of tissue for analysis. But as Susan later said, although he tried to explain all the reasons for his suggestion, once she heard the word *biopsy*, she stopped listening.

"I was terrified. I was so upset that when I came home I went to my room and couldn't eat or sleep for a week. Finally, my husband called the doctor, and he talked me into speaking with the physician again. I calmed myself and called the doctor, and he arranged to have the biopsy done the following day."

Susan's biopsy was negative. The anxiety had been of her own making. There was no basis for it.

"If I had had the presence of mind to listen to my doctor," she said, "I would have heard him say, 'It probably is not malignant, but I think we should rule out cancer.' I would have been able to sleep that night. But in my mind, I was convinced that he was keeping something from me."

She still shudders when she realizes that she had actually considered not having the biopsy done at all. "You know, of course, that I could still be sitting in that room of mine, terrified and depressed."

Susan's acute—and unnecessary—fear made her delay her biopsy for a week; the very thought of cancer can completely immobilize some people, with disastrous results.

Helen came from a large and caring European family. She was an outgoing, cheerful woman who often surprised neighbors with fresh-baked breads. Then one day she changed. She became distant and preferred to keep to herself. No one, not even her husband, was able to understand why Helen became a different person.

Eventually Helen not only stopped seeing people but also stopped eating. Finally she was hospitalized. Only then did she admit to having found a lump in her breast six months before. She said she knew it was cancer and couldn't bear to face it. She lived with the fear of the disease until she died from it a few months later.

Danielle did not make Helen's mistake. Her four children and her volunteer work left her little time to read, but she kept up with the news on television. Though not the type to worry about her health, Danielle was impressed by a report about breast self-examination. She learned the simple procedure and faithfully examined her breasts each month.

One day she discovered a lump. She went immediately to her doctor, whose response was, "Let's wait and see what develops." His easy-going manner and the fact that he did not suggest an immediate mammogram or biopsy set her mind to rest. She so trusted him that she never sought a second opinion. Ten months later, no second opinion was necessary. The tumor surfaced.

Danielle was hospitalized and had to undergo a radical mastectomy.

The story of Danielle enrages the women who hear it. Cases like this one make a woman wonder, "Whom can I trust?"

An informed woman can trust herself. She can trust her instincts. She can also trust her physician if she has chosen that physician carefully and thoughtfully. She will know what questions to ask and how to evaluate the answers.

WOMEN AND CANCER

This book is about cancer of the female reproductive system and breast: Nearly half of all cancers that affect women are concentrated in these sites.

Breast cancer is still the leading cause of death by cancer in America today. In 1980, it was estimated that more than 109,000 women would develop breast cancer. By 1981 that figure rose to 110,000, and by 1982 and beyond it is expected to go still higher. Almost 100,000 women will develop other cancers of the reproductive system. In addition, another 45,000 are developing carcinoma *in situ* (the earliest form of cancer) of the cervix. The other major cancers that affect women (and men, too) are lung cancer and cancer of the colon and rectum.

As recently as ten years ago, when a woman had cancer it was considered a deep, dark secret. Cancer was something that people just did not talk about. The very word caused fear—among friends and relatives of victims as well as among the victims themselves. Some families were shunned because one member was known to have cancer. It was as though cancer were highly contagious. Even on obituary pages cancer was rarely mentioned. Instead it would be reported that the deceased had died after "a long illness" or "a prolonged illness."

The unreasoning fear began to dissipate after two well-known women—Betty Ford, wife of former president Gerald Ford, and Happy Rockefeller, wife of former vice president Nelson Rockefeller—announced that they had undergone mastectomies because of cancer. This new openness has been immensely beneficial. After all, how can we deal with a problem unless we can discuss it?

With cancer there is much to discuss—and not all news is bad news. For example, advances in detection techniques make it possible to spot many female cancers at earlier, more easily treatable stages. The cure rate for some cancers of the reproductive tract is virtually 100 percent if they are discovered in an early, localized stage before it is invasive and has spread. New simple-to-use tests are making possible at-home detection of colon and rectal cancer. And breast cancer—the number-one threat to women—can now be detected early enough to permit local treatment instead of breast removal. Meanwhile, for those women who must undergo mastectomies, the art of breast reconstruction has progressed sufficiently to permit them to have new breasts if they wish.

In the past cancer had been made to look so fearsome, so horrible, so inexplicable, that many people threw up their hands and said, in effect, "Oh, it's hopeless. I'd rather not know. Besides, it's all a matter of chance."

It is *not* a matter of chance. Staying healthy is frequently a matter of *choice*. When you read the stories of women who survived cancer, you will see that their survival was a matter of faith. Sometimes it was an old-fashioned religious faith; sometimes it was faith in themselves, their physicians, and treatments that helped them to overcome the disease. In still other instances, their faith took the form of an overpowering will to live, a refusal to admit the possibility of defeat.

Even before facing cancer, and even if you never do, it is important to face yourself and your health. You must know your own body so well that you know about staying healthy, spotting symptoms, exploring all options and alternatives should cancer strike, and working with the doctor within you. Women who claim to be taking good care of themselves often are only caring for their bodies on the outside. The woman who says, "I eat well, sleep well, and exercise," and yet ignores Pap smears and breast self-exams is choosing to ignore preventive measures against cancer. If you choose to ignore these preventive measures, you are taking unnecessary risks with your health and your life. Lung cancer, for example, is nearly 100 percent preventable—it entails, however, the perseverance to give up smoking.

Not all cancer is preventable. But *all* cancers respond better to treatment when caught in the early stages. *The sooner cancer is detected, the better the body, with medical help, is able to ward off the attack.* The body itself is not only healthier when treatment starts, but it also responds better to modern medicine. So part of staying healthy should be to get regular check-ups by a good gynecologist, have regular Pap smears, and examine your breasts regularly.

Cancer was named by Hippocrates, the father of medicine. The Greek word for crab is *karkinos*, and Hippocrates named the disease we now call cancer because of the pincerlike projections that physicians noticed when they examined women with breast cancer. Of course, by the time the disease appeared in this form it was almost always fatal. As a result, doctors in ancient times thought cancer incurable. As recently as the 1950s Dr. Harry Green, a distinguished professor from Yale University School of Medicine, often told his students, "Cancer always kills. If you were cured of cancer, you can be certain that you did not have cancer. Cancer is fatal." Although this may have seemed true at the time, today we know it is false.

Cancer is the name given to a collection of malignant, fast-growing cells that have the ability to invade and destroy healthy tissues. It is a complex disease, one with over 100 different variations. There are, however, four main types of cancers:

Carcinomas. These are the most common; they usually originate in the lining of organs such as the ovaries and breasts and intestines.

Leukemias. These arise in the blood-forming system.

Lymphomas. These develop and spread in the lymph system.

Sarcomas. These are the rarest; they develop in muscles, bones, and inside other organs.

When cancer develops, it stifles healthy cells, preventing them from doing the jobs they must do to keep the body functioning. Within the center of each cell, there is a nucleus containing deoxyribonucleic acid (DNA). DNA acts like a computer program that tells cells how and when to reproduce themselves and when to stop. The cancer cell does not get the message to stop, or if it does, it ignores it. Instead of "clicking off," the cancer cell defiantly continues to reproduce. In the normal life of cells, there is birth, maturity, and death, but cancer cells do not mature and die. They defiantly reproduce and reproduce and reproduce.

One of the many mysteries of cancer is why the body's defense system is not able to check the continued reproduction of cancer cells. In the normal, healthy body, the immune system fights off invaders. The immune system fights viruses and, in theory, should attack cancers, too. Cancer cells, however, seem to have the ability to disguise themselves so as to escape detection. One of the latest attempts to explain this is called the cocoon theory, which was suggested in 1979 by a team of researchers at Massachusetts General Hospital. In studies with guinea pigs, the researchers found that tumors secreted a substance called fibrin gel that covered them, apparently protecting them from the body's defense system.

You might think of the cancer cell as someone who has moved into your house and then decided there isn't enough room. Rather than pack up and go home, the visitor decides to expand, first into other rooms in your house and then into your next-door neighbor's house as well. If left unchecked, the cancerous invader will keep expanding and eventually move to distant sites.

As cancer reproduces, it proceeds through three main stages. They are preinvasive, invasive, and metastatic.

Preinvasive

The earliest state of cancer is called the preinvasive or *in situ* stage. Here cells have reproduced abnormally and have acquired abnormal properties, but they are still in the tissue in which they originated. All cancers respond best to treatment when caught in the preinvasive stages. Early cases of carcinoma *in situ* of the cervix, the vulva, and the endometrium (the lining of the uterus) are nearly 100 percent curable.

Invasive

From the preinvasive stage, if the cancer progresses, it makes inroads in the local tissue; that is, it pushes other cells out of its way. When this happens, it is said to be in the invasive stage.

If the cancer is caught early in the invasive stage, chances of a cure are still good. According to the American Cancer Society (ACS), the five-year survival rate for women whose cancer is detected at the earliest stage is 85 percent in the case of cancers of the breast, 86 percent for the endometrium, and 78 percent in the case of cervical cancer.

If the cancer, though still localized, has progressed further in the invasive stage before it is detected and treated, then the chances of a cure diminish. For the later invasive stages, ACS statistics show five-year survival rates of 47 percent for breast cancer, 37 percent for cervical cancer, and 33 percent for cancer of the uterus and endometrium.

Metastatic

When cancer cells have spread to sites different from their origin, cancer is said to have metastasized. Cells have shot off from the original tumor and been carried through the blood and lymph systems to remote parts. This stage of cancer is usually not curable. There are, however, cases of women who have survived many years after the diagnosis of metastases, frequently while leading active and normal lives. Progress in treatment provides daily proof of the power of modern medicine in these cases.

THE CAUSES OF CANCER

Cancer seems to have many causes. A normal cell might be transformed into a malignant one as a result of viruses, radiation, and chemicals such as certain food additives.

In addition to cancer causes, there are cancer promoters. A promoter might be a food, a chemical, or an environmental condition that enhances your chances for developing cancer. A predisposition to cancer may also be inherited.

Environmental factors and diet seem to be very important. Testimony at hearings conducted by Senator George McGovern's Select Committee on Nutrition in 1977 suggested that nearly 70 percent of all cancers are environmentally related and that diet plays a crucial role in encouraging the disease. The importance of diet also was stressed by Dr. Diane Fink, coordinator of the Diet, Nutrition, and Cancer Program of the National Cancer Institute, who was quoted in the December 14, 1979, issue of the *Journal of the American Medical Association* as saying that "we believe there are enough data to suggest that diet is a factor in causing cancer, particularly breast, colon, and endometrial cancer." In case of breast and endometrial cancer, a number of studies indicate that the true dietary culprit may be fat.

Other forms of cancer seem to have other causes. Cervical cancer, for example, is now often described as "a viral-related cancer" because of its frequent association with the genital herpes virus. Herpes virus itself is usually sexually transmitted, so cervical cancer may also be a related venereal disease.

Vaginal cancers and even cancer of the vulva are thought to be caused by outside agents. Women exposed to certain agricultural chemicals may be at greater risk for developing vulvar cancer. Women exposed before birth to the synthetic hormone DES have been found to have a high incidence of vaginal cancer. We will discuss the causes of each type of cancer in detail in the following chapters.

Cancer seems to strike wantonly, but when we look at its causes, we can see that in many cases the disease is *preventable, treatable,* and *curable.* The crucial factor in the success of treatment, however, is still early detection. And prevention, of course, is better yet.

Chapter Two

Preventing and Conquering Cancer

Alicia was twenty-eight when she was hospitalized for severe stomach pains. During exploratory surgery, her physician discovered a mass in her pelvis. Alicia had ovarian cancer. Her physician had just learned of a new drug and the hospital had access to it. Some of its known side effects were devastating: It poisoned the bone marrow and actually stopped blood production. It was, however, also thought to be a somewhat effective treatment for ovarian cancer.

Alicia weighed the risks and the benefits. She knew that without the drug, her chances for surviving were almost *nil*. But even with the drug, she might not survive.

Alicia so wanted to live, however, that she took the gamble. She put complete faith in the physician treating her and decided to try the drug. That was twenty-two years ago, and she is still alive.

Alicia was, in fact, one of the first patients in the United States to undergo chemotherapy (chemical or drug treatment) specifically for cancer of the reproductive organs. In her case the cure took several steps. In addition to the chemotherapy, Alicia had three operations in three years. Today, such combination treatments are being hailed as the most promising way to cure cancer.

Although the combined therapies of surgery and radiation and/or chemotherapy are used effectively in many types of cancer, the most dependable and promising results have come about in the area of cancer of the reproductive systems. The response rate—meaning the percentage of patients in whom cancer has been significantly diminished—has doubled for ovarian cancer, which was first considered treatable some twenty years ago.

For Alicia, conquering cancer has been a victory on many levels. When she first learned she had cancer, the emotional strain was so severe that she lost her job. Then her marriage ended in a messy divorce. But within five years, after her initial surgery and chemotherapy treatment, she had found not only a better job but a new man as well. Alicia soon remarried and felt secure enough to move to a suburb of New York, a full hour away from the hospital where she still receives her chemotherapy injections each month. The once-a-month hospital visit does not interfere with Alicia's busy social schedule. She is grateful to be alive. She finds being close to fifty very satisfying. "I will never complain about my age," she says. "When I am ninety, I will still feel like a woman reborn."

Ask Alicia the question, "Is cancer curable?" and she will be quick to answer, "Yes." In medical circles, however, the word *cure* is a highly controversial one. As journalist-physician Lawrence K. Altman reported in a *New York Times* article, most doctors feel *cure* is too absolute a term. They are more comfortable using phrases like "no evidence of disease" or "long-term survival." "We want to cure cancer in your lifetime" is the slogan, nonetheless, of the American Cancer Society.

Despite the cautious attitude of doctors, treatments for cancer have so improved in terms of surgery, radiation, and chemotherapy that many more physicians are now talking about cure rates, as opposed to response rates. A cure rate generally is expressed in terms of the percentage of patients free of cancer five years after diagnosis. Doctors are more likely to talk about cure rates when the disease is caught in the earliest stage.

Because early-detection methods are so readily available, treatments are so improved, and the cure rates are so much better than they were ten years ago, we want you to see that today cancer is conquerable.

If you do develop cancer, you should find the best doctors and best treatments for your particular case (see pp.). The standard treatments for cancer today are surgery, chemotherapy, and radiation. The treatments are not always pleasant, but neither are they always devastating. We know of women being treated for cancer today who have not let the disease interfere with their lives. (We will discuss each treatment, as well as its physical and emotional side effects, in a separate chapter.) We stress that the sooner cancer is detected, the better your chances for long-term survival and minimal treatments. For those of you who have seen friends become ill due to chemotherapy and have wondered, "Is it worth it," we ask you to remember Alicia's story. She gambled on life and won!

Many women are alive today because they took a chance on treatment. Many more will be alive tomorrow, if they make the choice now to become informed.

BEING INFORMED

Being an informed woman means that you know your own medical history at least as well as your physician does. In most instances, your internist will have a complete chart recording your medical and family history.

An internist is a doctor of internal medicine who treats a variety of illnesses. He or she may treat for sore throats, ulcers, arthritis, and a wide range of other related and unrelated illnesses. Today the internist has largely replaced the general practitioner or family

YOUR MEDICAL HISTORY

Name______________ Age____ Sex_______ Date__________

FAMILY HISTORY	*Age today*	*State of health*	*If deceased, cause of death and age at death*
Father	____	____	________
Mother	____	____	________
Brothers	____	____	________
	____	____	________
Sisters	____	____	________
	____	____	________

FAMILY ILLNESSES Alcoholism, allergy, arthritis, benign tumors, (e.g., fibroids), bleeding, *cancer, *diabetes, epilepsy, heart disease, high blood pressure, kidney trouble, lung disease, mental illness, stroke, thyroid disease, any other disease not listed______________

____

PERSONAL HISTORY Country of birth:__________

Foreign travel:__________

Weight:______ *Recent change:__________

Habits: *Diet, alcohol, coffee, exercise, medicines, sleep, *tobacco______

SOCIAL HISTORY Marital status________ Children_______

Health of spouse and children__________

Occupations, past and present__________

*Environmental exposures__________

Hobbies and interests__________

ACUTE INFECTIONS Chicken pox, diptheria, hepatitis, malaria, measles, meningitis, mononucleosis, *mumps, polio, rheumatic fever, scarlet fever, tuberculosis, whooping cough, other, *herpes virus (cold sores of mouth or vulva)__________

ALLERGIES: Asthma, drugs, hay fever, hives__________

ALLERGY INJECTIONS__________

BLOOD COUNTS (and results of tests for cholesterol levels and triglycerides)

____

SURGERY AND DATES__________

INJURIES AND DATES__________

*X-RAY TREATMENTS AND DATES__________

IMMUNIZATIONS Diptheria, polio, smallpox, tetanus, rubella, rubeola, other

____

HEAD Concussion, headache__________

EYES Glaucoma, infection, vision disturbance________________

EARS Infection, hearing trouble________________

NOSE Bleeding, congestion, sinus infection________________

MOUTH AND THROAT Dental disease, hoarseness, sore throats, tonsillitis ________________

RESPIRATORY SYSTEM Blood coughed up, bronchitis, cough, phlegm, pneumonia, *tuberculosis________________

HEART Chest pain, heart murmur, *high blood pressure, swelling of feet, pressure, shortness of breath after exertion or in middle of night________________

*BREASTS Cysts, pain, swelling, tumor________________

VASCULAR SYSTEM Leg pain, phlebitis, varicose veins, cold hands and feet ________________

STOMACH AND INTESTINES Bleeding, burning, diarrhea, constipation, food intolerance, gas, hermorrhoids, indigestion, nausea, pain, poor appetite, rectal pain, ulcer, vomiting________________

LIVER AND GALLBLADDER Gallstones, jaundice, fatty food intolerance ________________

URINARY SYSTEM Bleeding, cystitis, difficulty holding urine, frequency of urination, infection, kidney stones, pain________________

*MENSTRUAL HISTORY Age started ( ), length of cycle ( ), cramps, days of flow ( ), heavy or irregular periods, last menstrual period________________

*SEXUAL EXPERIENCE Age at first sexual intercourse ( )

*PREGNANCIES Number ( ), miscarriages ( ), births ( ), age at first pregnancy ( ), age at first childbirth ( ), complications, natural deliveries or cesarean, if cesarean, indicate why________________

*BIRTH CONTROL Method________________

*VAGINAL AND/OR PELVIC INFECTIONS Burning, discharge, itching ________________

NEUROLOGIC SYSTEM Dizziness, fainting, numbness, paralysis, seizures, stroke________________

EMOTIONAL HISTORY Anxiety, depression, insomnia, tension________________

METABOLIC SYSTEM Diabetes, gout, other________________

ENDOCRINE SYSTEM Thyroid, adrenal________________

SKIN Cysts, infection, rash________________

BLOOD Anemia, bleeding, transfusion________________

BONES, JOINTS Arthritis, bone disease________________

ADDITIONAL INFORMATION________________

____

____

____

doctor. If, instead of an internist, your obstetrician-gynecologist is your primary physician, you should ask him or her to check your blood pressure and listen to your heart and lungs, as well as performing the general gynecological exam (which includes a breast and pelvic exam).

When your obstetrician-gynecologist is your primary-care physician, you might have a slight advantage over those women seeing internists when it comes to determining female cancers. The obstetrician-gynecologist will have more experience in seeing and treating female cancers simply because it is his or her specialty. Keep in mind, however, that an internist is most concerned with your overall medical condition. Regardless of the kind of physician you are seeing, ask whether a chart on you exists. If it doesn't, have your doctor make a chart for you or make your own.

Even if there is a medical record in your physician's office, you should know your own medical history. The following chart is a sample of what you should know about yourself. The most important sections in terms of female cancers are starred. On this chart, you may fill in or circle the information as it applies to you. The section marked "Additional information" can be used to expand upon anything in the chart or to add other relevant information.

The physician who takes a good history—yours and your family's—is offering you one of the first and most important preventive steps to take against cancer. Some diseases follow such a definite pattern that the family history might enable your doctor to tell whether or not you are at high risk and what you can do to prevent yourself from becoming a cancer statistic. Some cancers, such as breast cancer, do run in families. Some inherent family conditions, such as obesity, might put you in a high-risk category for endometrial cancer.

If the doctor you are seeing has not asked you some of the questions listed on the chart and you feel they are important, jot down a list of them yourself and bring them with you on your next visit. If your doctor gives you a wave of the hand that means, "You are being ridiculous," wave yourself right out of his or her office and find yourself another physician.

If there are questions on this chart that you cannot answer, begin by calling your relatives. If your mother is alive, ask her, and ask your sisters, your aunts, and anyone else who can help—even physicians whom you have seen in the past.

If you are adopted, call an organization involved with adopted persons' rights to get a copy of your *natural* mother's medical history or cause of death if she is deceased. Knowing your medical history is the first step.

FINDING A PHYSICIAN

An entire book can be written on this topic alone. How do you find a doctor? Most of us ask a friend. Some of us ask other physicians. Sometimes we choose a doctor just because he or she happens to be in a convenient area. It is important that you have a gynecologist whom you consider highly competent and qualified to give you routine exams and who will be aware in your middle years of any signs and symptoms that might indicate early cancers.

What is it that you should look for in a physician? In general, if you are looking for a gynecologist and/or obstetrician-gynecologist, you will want someone with a hospital affiliation who has a well-run office.

If you need a physician and don't have referral suggestions from doctors or knowledgeable friends, then call the director of obstetrics and gynecology at a major teaching hospital in your area, or contact your local medical society and ask for a list of names of the specialists in the field. Then it is up to you to find out which of these physicians is best for you. Ask friends, relatives, business associates, anyone you can. Check to see whether any of the candidates on your list have written articles in medical journals or the popular press; perhaps these will give you some hint as to the type of interests they have.

After compiling a list of physicians, Isadore Rosenfeld, M.D., author of *The Complete Medical Exam* and *Second Opinion*, says, "Interview them." Just because your friends may have liked a doctor does not necessarily mean that you will. Call the physician's office and tell the nurse that you would like about ten minutes to talk with the doctor, to see whether he or she is interested in you and your particular family history or problems, and to find out whether you get along well. What happens if, after the interview, you don't like the doctor? Go elsewhere. Why invest your time, your money, and your blood with someone with whom you don't feel comfortable?

What will it cost to interview a doctor? Ask the nurse what the fee is for an initial visit and examination, and approximately how long it will take. Then figure a consultation should cost you about half that. You might ask whether there is a set consultation fee. In some rare instances, the doctor won't charge for an interview. Most will, however, charge a full fee. After talking with the physician and determining his or her interest and areas of specialization (even gynecologists today specialize), if you are pleased, make an appointment for an examination at some other time.

When you are dealing with your body, there are enough good physicians available for you to afford to be choosy. Don't be stuck with someone whom you dislike just because you think he or she is good. Try to choose a doctor who is not only technically expert but caring as well. Since your emotions and your body may not require the same attention, however, keep technical proficiency high on your list. Above all, you want someone you can trust.

It is especially important that you choose a physician who allows you to ask questions and who answers them. The more your physician tells you about your treatments—cancer treatments especially—the less likely that you will be frightened.

What happens when a physician about whom you have heard rave reviews and whom you have interviewed begins to treat you coldly and indifferently? This is a difficult question to answer. It may be that you should examine your attitude as well as the doctor's. We know of one arrogant woman who needed only a few seconds to turn a kindly, caring physician into an ogre. Her behavior might not have mattered if he had not just had an argument with his wife on the telephone. Doctors are human, too.

A young Boston mother went to a physician whom she had seen once before. On her second visit he was distant and unresponsive and appeared to be rushing her.

"Thoroughly disgusted with him, I got up to walk out," she said. "Something stopped me. I looked at him and said, 'Doctor, you were so pleasant the first time I saw you that I'm afraid I am rather confused by your attitude today. I hope nothing is wrong.'

"Well, you can imagine my surprise," she continued, "when he replied, 'Yes, something is wrong. I am trying to rush out of here to get to the hospital. A little girl I was treating has suddenly gone into a coma. I gave her parents every reason to believe we had her cancer licked. Can you imagine how they must feel right now?'"

"Yes, I can," answered the woman. "My sister-in-law lost a child this week."

The rapport established, the physician told the woman he would phone her that evening, and he did.

CHOOSING SPECIALISTS AND HOSPITALS

The first decision for a person stricken with cancer is where to go for treatment—to what kind of doctor and at what kind of hospital? Does one go to a physician who specializes in tumors or to a physician who is a specialist in the particular part of the body that has been afflicted? Does one go to whatever hospital is nearest or to one of the nation's major medical teaching hospitals or cancer centers?

No hard-and-fast answers can be given to these questions. Even among doctors there is debate as to which kind of physician is most qualified to treat the cancer patient. In practice, of course, with a disease such as cancer, frequently more than one physician will be involved in treating a case.

The physician who specializes in tumors is called an oncologist. Oncology is the study of cancer—the study of new growths of abnormal cells and how they affect the body. It is a relatively new specialty in the United States and not many physicians have received formal training in oncology during the past twenty years. A gynecologist oncologist is a specialist in female cancers. You might choose to use one for your routine exams, but this would usually be impractical.

How would you go about finding a gynecologic oncologist? Usually they are affiliated with comprehensive cancer centers or teaching hospitals, and you will be referred to one by your own physician. For rare types of cancer, even gynecologic oncologists might specialize; ask what types of cancers they treat most often.

Obviously it is at the major teaching hospitals and cancer centers shat you will find the most sophisticated equipment, the most advanced treatments, and the best-trained personnel. For a list of them, see Appendix A.

To encourage hospitals to continually improve their anti-cancer efforts, the American College of Surgeons evaluates hospital-based cancer programs. According to its *Cancer Program Manual,* the ACS's Commission on Cancer is attempting to "encourage each hospital or institution to improve its cancer control efforts in the areas of prevention, early diagnosis, pretreatment evaluation, staging, optimal treatment, rehabilitation, surveillance for recurrent and multiple primary cancer, and care of dying patients." For a number of years, ACS used a I, II, III or S rating system on its list of approved cancer programs. It now breaks the programs down into six categories. The Cancer Treatment Comprehensive Program means that at least 85 percent of the institution's caseload consists of cancer patients. It offers a full range of services for diagnosis and treatment, and its staff includes members of all specialties. It also provides post-graduate residencies in oncology. A Teaching Hospital Cancer Program provides the same services, except for the post-graduate training. A Community Hospital Comprehensive Program, which handles over 300 new cases of cancer per year, differs primarily in that it may not offer a complete range of treatments and you may have to be referred elsewhere. A Community Hospital Cancer Program handles fewer patients—over 100 new cases per year. A Special Cancer Program is for the diagnosis and treatment of a specific type of cancer (in a pediatric hospital, for example).

Some people with cancer may also wish to contribute to the struggle to find a cure for it by participating in one of the study groups in the National Cancer Institute's (NCI) Cancer Therapy Evaluation Program. A person's local physician can make arrangements for participation. In some cases, patients participating in the NCI-funded groups will be treated without cost. Not everyone who wishes will necessarily be admitted to a study group. Members must fit the particular needs of a group and often consent to experimental treatments. Sometimes a patient may qualify for a group but find it is a great distance from his or her home. Still, study groups are useful and helpful. Your physician can check the details for you.

The study groups are divided by region and by particular kinds of cancer. For a current list of the groups and their chairpersons, you should contact National Cancer Institute directly (see Appendix C) or your gynecologic-oncologist. These groups change frequently.

Being in the best hospital does not necessarily mean you are going to get the best care. Whatever the size of the hospital, the important thing is to be able to stay on top of the course of treatment that you and your physician decide is best. This is true whether you are hospitalized to have surgery on an ingrown toenail or to have a breast removed.

Despite the advantages of large institutions, many women will choose to be treated at a small community hospital. There the faces are often friendlier. Some women have said they are afraid that at the major teaching centers they will be used as experimental guinea pigs or that doctors will do everything in their power to keep them alive even if their cases are terminal and they are in great pain.

In the end, the patient probably will decide on the basis of what feels most comfortable to her. Some people have implicit faith in their family doctor,whom they have known for perhaps thirty years. They believe the doctor "knows best": If the family doctor says the hospital down the street is the place to go, that is where they will go. Other people will react differently; they will check different hospitals and interview a host of doctors, looking for the one with the best credentials, the most sympathetic personality, or the greatest willingness to explain every detail to them.

We place a great deal of importance on finding and seeking out the right physician. This is not an easy task, but we do not mean to make it sound like an insurmountable one. Finding a good physician and discovering who it is who has what drugs available might well bring you to roadblocks, detours, hurdles, and pitfalls. But it is worth jumping hurdles to find the physician who is best for you.

Chapter Three

The Cervix

Patrice left Manhattan for the suburbs after giving birth to her second child. Because she considered herself to be a "city girl," she never lost touch with her friends in Manhattan. Although she found a suburban pediatrician for her daughters, she continued using the same New York obstetrician who had delivered her babies for her own routine check-ups. As her daughters grew older and became involved in school activities, they took more and more of Patrice's time. When they were ages six and seven, she realized she had not had a breast examination or Pap test (used to detect cervical cancer) in three years.

Finally Patrice's uncle, himself a physician, found her a doctor near her home; she referred to this man as "the local hick." Said Patrice, "I went to him because I figured, how far wrong could someone go on a breast exam and a Pap test?"

Two weeks after her check-up, Patrice's Pap test came back with a report of Class 3—abnormal cells, possibly cancerous. Patrice panicked. Her uncle panicked. The local physician hospitalized Patrice, gave her a D and C (dilation and curettage), and told her she was fine.

Even though the story appears to have a happy ending, Patrice's ordeal may have been unnecessary. Hospitalization should have occurred only after an office biopsy showed some definite abnormal cell changes. If Patrice had sought a second opinion, or if she had gone to a specialist initially, or even if she had been admitted to a teaching hospital, she would have been given a second Pap test to confirm the results of the first. If the second Pap test also showed abnormalities, she would then have had a colposcopic exam, which involves the use of a specially designed microscope to look at the cells of the cervix. If the colposcopy showed abnormal cell changes relating to an early cancer, and this was confirmed by biopsy, then and only then would she have been given further treatment.

Many women go through abnormal Pap smear scares, and most are treated effectively. Patrice's treatment is somewhat unusual in this day and age. Physicians, whether in cities or in suburbs, most often are following standardized procedures. Patrice never questioned her physician; she just followed orders.

What *should* happen in the event of a Class 3 Pap test report is best seen in the story of Nora.

Before her marriage, Nora worked for a state attorney general. Nora had no law degree or formal training, but she was multilingual, efficient, and a workaholic. She had such a knack for organization that she planned election campaigns and directed the placement of legal staff throughout the state.

After her marriage, Nora combined her full-time career with her commitment to being the perfect super-wife. To maintain her busy schedule she began to cut back on visits with friends, trips to the hairdresser, and shopping sprees. Then she decided that her regular check-up for her Pap test and breast examination would have to wait a bit. Two years lapsed between visits.

When Nora told one of the campaign workers about her cutbacks, her friend said, "Nora, you owe yourself the luxury of good health." Nora decided to make the time to see her doctor.

In the past Nora had always had perfectly normal Pap test ratings, but this time the Pap test was Class 3, abnormal cells present. She had a repeat Pap smear; this, too, was a Class 3. The physician performed a colposcopic exam, then took a small biopsy, and from the diagnosis told Nora she had carcinoma *in situ*, the earliest form of cancer of the cervix.

Nora was hospitalized and treated by conization. This procedure, which involves taking a cone-shaped piece of tissue from the cervix, is used both diagnostically to confirm the presence of abnormal cells and therapeutically as a treatment for very early forms of cancer.

Every three months for two years afterward Nora returned to her physician for Pap smears and colposcopic exams to make certain that there was no recurrence of abnormal cells. For two years Nora was fine. Then she conceived, and during her pregnancy Pap smears again showed signs of carcinoma *in situ*, which were treated with a repeat conization. Nora gave birth, nonetheless, to a normal, healthy child.

Since her pregnancy Nora's case has been followed very closely. If the carcinoma *in situ* again returns, she may need another cone biopsy. But with this procedure she is able to keep her cervix, keep her uterus, and still have the option of having another child.

When carcinoma *in situ* is diagnosed, women who want children generally will choose minimal treatment. In fact, women past their reproductive years sometimes choose minimal treatment also. But when carcinoma *in situ* returns, even just once after an initial attack, physicians frequently suggest removal of the cervix and uterus.

Deciding which treatment for this preinvasive cancer is best for you can be difficult. Many women prefer treatments that permit them to retain all their reproductive organs. Other women feel safer without a cervix that may give them recurring problems. All women should realize that there is a choice in treatment when abnormal cell changes of the cervix are detected early.

It is expected that in 1981 approximately 16,000 cases of invasive cancer of the cervix will be detected. For about half the women diagnosed, the disease will be fatal. It is important to remember that even invasive cancer is treatable and, in some cases, curable. In addition to invasive cancer, there will be an estimated 45,000 new cases of carcinoma *in situ* detected. Carcinoma *in situ* has a near-perfect cure rate.

Cervical cancer will be detected in fifteen of every 100,000 white women in the United States and in about thirty-four of every 100,000 black women. Any woman can develop cervical cancer, even a woman who does not fit the high-risk profile. With cervical cancer, however, some women are at greater risk than others. Women who have had early and frequent sex have a greater chance for developing the disease than women who are celibate. One theory is that cervical cancer is caused by a virus transmitted through sexual intercourse. This theory is based on the observation that cervical cancer is most frequently detected in prostitutes, whereas nuns do not seem to develop cervical cancer.

In her book *You Can Fight Cancer and Win, New York Times* columnist Jane Brody discusses "what cancer is not caused by." She says that cervical cancer "is not 'just desserts' for moral turpitude; rather it is associated with sexual activity, which most of us engage in from time to time."

No one really knows for certain what constitutes the "early and frequent sex" with many partners that plays a role in cervical cancer. Intuitively, the young teens (thirteen to fifteen) seem early, but it is impossible to say whether "many" means three, five, or seven partners in one night, one week, one month, one year, or one lifetime. Theoretically, if the disease is transmitted through the male, then the more partners one has, the greater the chance one has of getting it. At the same time, it also has to be remembered that some women developed cervical cancer even though they *never* had sexual intercourse.

It has also been observed that women who have had genital herpes infections, specifically the virus called HVH-2 *(herpes virus hominis)*, are at greater risk of developing cervical cancer. Because it can be transmitted through sexual intercourse, the virus is classed as a venereal disease. Genital herpes was once thought to be a disease of the poorer classes, but if this was ever so, it is certainly not true any longer. The incidence of the disease has been increasing rapidly in all income groups in recent years. It appears that women who have had carcinoma *in situ* of the cervix are more likely to have herpes antibodies in their blood, showing that they have this disease (genital herpes), than women who have never had carcinoma *in situ*. This association gives collateral support to the theory that cervical cancer might be linked with the herpes virus or some other infectious organism.

Another theory is that cervical cancer is caused or promoted by some components of smegma—a substance secreted by the sebaceous glands that collects under the foreskin of the penis. This theory, also unproven, is based on the observation that the incidence of cervical cancer seems to be especially low in Jewish and Moslem societies, where male babies are routinely circumcized.

WHAT IS THE CERVIX?

The cervix is the neck of the uterus or womb. If you imagine your uterus as an upside-down pear, which is what it really looks like, then the cervix would be the narrow end that extends slightly into the upper part of your vagina. The uterus itself is high inside your body, out of reach. The cervix, however, which is shaped like a short cylinder and is attached to the uterus and to the circumference of your vagina, extends into the vagina just far enough for you to be able to touch it.

The cervix is tiny, only about one inch long and one inch in diameter, but it plays several important roles. It is through the cervix that menstrual blood flows. It is also through the tiny cervix

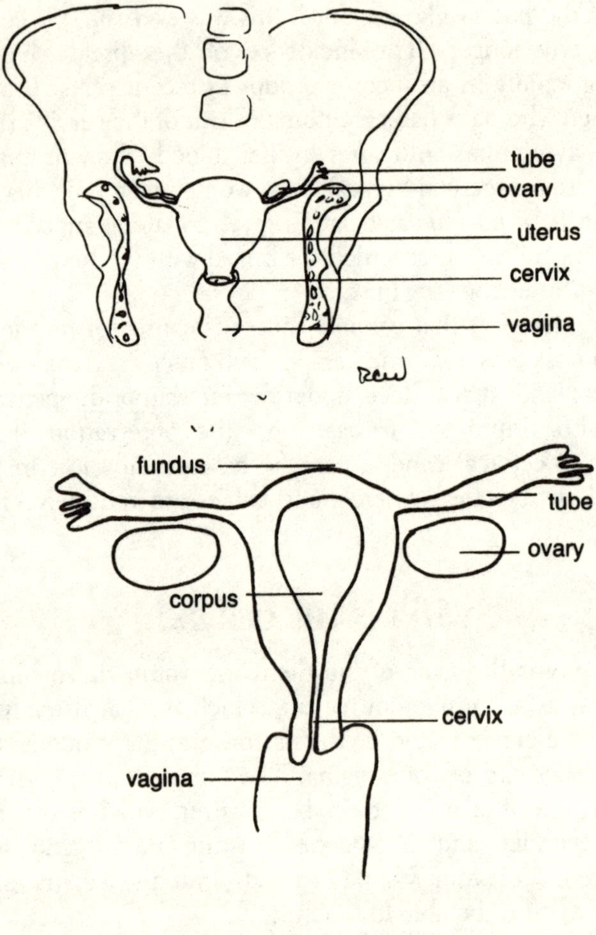

The pelvis and internal genitalia. Top figure shows the location of the internal genitalia within the pelvic girdle. Bottom figure gives a clearer view of the organs.

that the entire body of a new baby will pass during childbirth. If the cervical gate does not open sufficiently, a cesarean delivery will be necessary.

In addition, the cervix plays a vital role in the conception of a child. During intercourse, sperm can pass readily and easily through the canal of the cervix if the time of the reproductive cycle is right. The slippery, clear, jellylike mucus secreted by the cervix assists the sperm in making their way toward the ovaries. If the sperm entering the cervix eventually finds an egg and fertilizes it, the os, the mouth of the cervix, shuts itself up tightly with a plug of modified mucus that remains in place until the end of pregnancy.

When examining your cervix your physician will use a speculum, a duckbill-shaped instrument that spreads the walls of your vagina. If you have never had children, when the physician looks at your cervix he or she will see a small shining pink dome with a tiny opening—the os—in the center. The mouth of the cervix looks like a tiny slit; it is no bigger than the end of a cotton swab stick. This condition is called being *nulliparous*, which means no children. If you have been pregnant and given birth, your cervical opening will be wider and rippled. This is called being *multiparous*, which means many children or pregnancies. It might also be referred to as *parous*, which simply means having been pregnant.

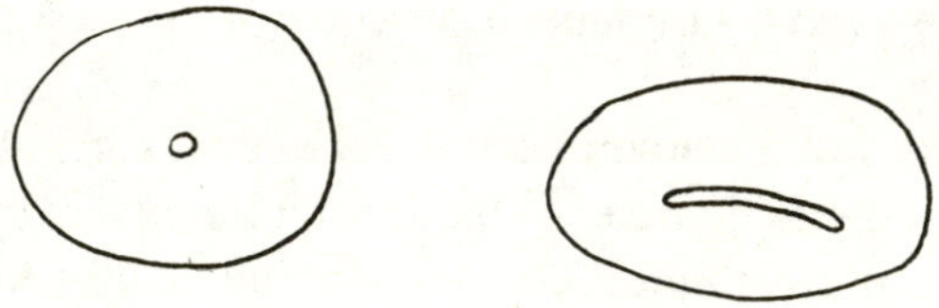

The cervix. At the left is the cervix of a nulliparous woman—one who has had no children. At right is the cervix of a multiparous woman—one who has had one or more completed pregnancies.

It is difficult to see your own cervix, but not impossible. With a plastic speculum (obtainable from many women's health organizations) and a mirror, you will be able to see it. Most women, however, find that it is much easier to feel the cervix than to see it. You can feel your cervix with your middle finger if you elevate one leg slightly or rest it on a chair and bend forward a bit, or you might prefer a squatting position.

Women who regularly examine their cervix do become attuned to its changes. Usually the cervix is as hard as the tip of your nose. Around the time of menstruation, it becomes somewhat softer in texture. At midcycle it feels so soft that you might be able to depress it slightly around the os, and it may also feel sticky because it secretes more mucus than usual. Just before the time of ovulation the mucus is cloudy, white, and thick. At the time of ovulation the mucus becomes slippery and clear (like the white of a raw egg), and it can be stretched in long threads between your fingers.

Because changes in cervical mucus can be so pronounced, women have long used the cervix as a fertility indicator. Evelyn and John Billings, two Australian doctors, have devised a method of natural birth control through cervical mucus tests that women are using today with varying degrees of success. It is described in their book, *Atlas of the Ovulation Method*, published by The Liturgical Press in 1974. Some women report using this method for years without a slip-up. But for many medical and technical reasons, most women should not depend on cervical indications alone as a fertility index.

Whether or not a woman examines her own cervix to determine fertility is not the issue here. What is important is that women who want to learn more about themselves should be able to understand the workings of the cervix during its normal healthy state. If you are familiar with your body as it looks and feels when it is well, you are more likely to notice the vaginal and vulvar changes that come about with certain types of cancers and infections. It is because so many women were told, "Don't touch yourself *there*," while they were growing up that more than half the cases of vulvar and vaginal cancers today are detected too late for optimal treatment.

THE CELLS OF THE CERVIX

The cervix is covered by a smooth *epithelium* (skin). It is pinkish-gray in color because of the way light reflects off the many cell layers with their underlying red blood supply.

The cells near the surface of the cervix are usually flat shinglelike cells called *squames*. They resemble the skin cells on the face, back, neck, hands, and other parts of the body. This tissue is also called *squamous epithelium*; cases of cancer of the cervix are somtimes referred to as *squamous cell carcinoma*. The squamous epithelium is a protective covering. If you think of what happens to the dead skin that we sometimes find leaving our bodies after a bath, you will understand how the uppermost layer of the cervix functions; it is shed and replaced by other living cells that have matured directly beneath the top layer of old ones and then move to the surface. This is a normal situation that happens all the time (see page 34 for illustration).

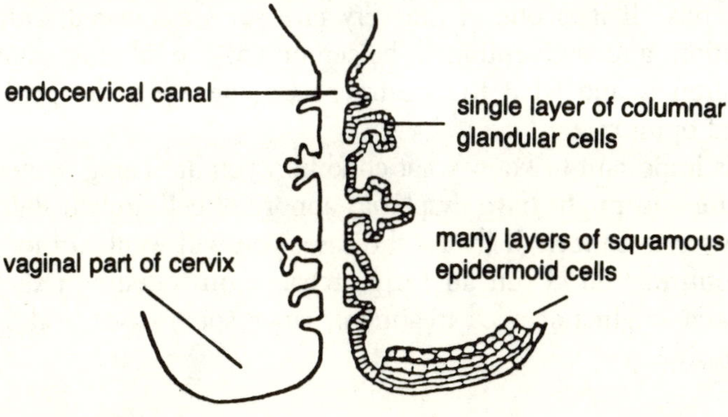

The lining of the cervix.

The inner canal of the cervix has columnar cells that under the microscope look like small tubes lined up side by side in a single layer or row. It is these columnar cells that secrete the cervical mucus.

Columnar cells are translucent, but they are only a single layer deep and so appear to be quite red because of the underlying blood vessels. For years physicians called this red area an "erosion of the cervix." After a pregnancy, women talking to other women could be overheard saying, "Since that last child of mine, half of my cervix has been eaten out—eroded." In fact, this is a misnomer. True "erosions" are like ulcers on the cervix, but they are rare. They occur primarily with syphilis, tuberculosis, herpes virus infections, cancer, or streptococci infections.

Some books for women and even some physicians today still refer to cervical erosions or "sores." They suggest that in severe or chronic cases of cervicitis (inflammation of the cervix) an inflamed area can be seen on the cervix which they will treat by cauterizing.

If a physician tells you that you are being treated for erosions, insist that he or she tell you exactly what condition exists. If it is ectropion, it requires *no* treatment. Ectropion is not a disease; it is the spread of normal columnar-secreting cells on to the surface of the cervix. If it is one of the very rare sores associated with the conditions already mentioned, be certain you are told just what the condition is and what the treatment will be. Consider getting a second opinion.

It is important to know what condition you are being treated for because you might have dysplasia, abnormal cell growth that is a precursor to cancer. If that is the case, you will want further tests for confirmation. Even an early precancerous condition such as dysplasia might not need treatment, since some cases heal spontaneously.

THE T ZONE: WHERE CANCER BEGINS

Between the outer squamous epithelium and the inner columnar cells is a microscopic area called the T zone: the transition or transformation zone. The T zone is the junction between the two kinds of cells (outer and inner), and it is in this area that most cancer precursors and cancers start. The zone may be limited to the narrow region just at the os, or it may spread over the outer part of the cervix. When a Pap smear is taken, the physician collects cells to be analyzed from the T zone. In some women the transition zone extends well into the outermost part of the cervix. So instead of an area covered primarily with grayish pearly squamous epithelium, they have a wide area covered with columnar cells that have spread down from the internal canal.

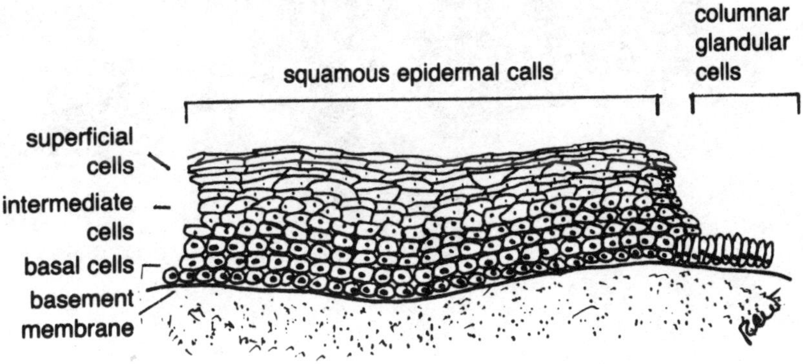

The T-Zone. This transition or transformation zone is the junction between the outer squamous epithelium and the inner columnar cells. The squamous cells are at left (mature cells are on top; newer cells underneath). Columnar glandular cells are at right.

Why is this T zone the site of cancer? Is it a more susceptible area? At the moment, no one knows for sure. In the normal cervix there is an orderly arrangement of squamous epithelium. The older shinglelike cells form the top layer, and the newer, rounder cells with large centers (nuclei) lie beneath. With dysplasia the orderly progression becomes disrupted, and the younger cells with the larger centers can be seen moving to the top.

With invasive cancer, cells are totally disarranged. Those that should be on the surface have pushed their way into the inner regions of the cervix. These cells can cluster together to form a tumor and then shoot off other cells that invade the inner tissues of the cervix, the nerves, the blood, and the lymph system. Once in the lymph or blood system, cancer travels to other parts of the body.

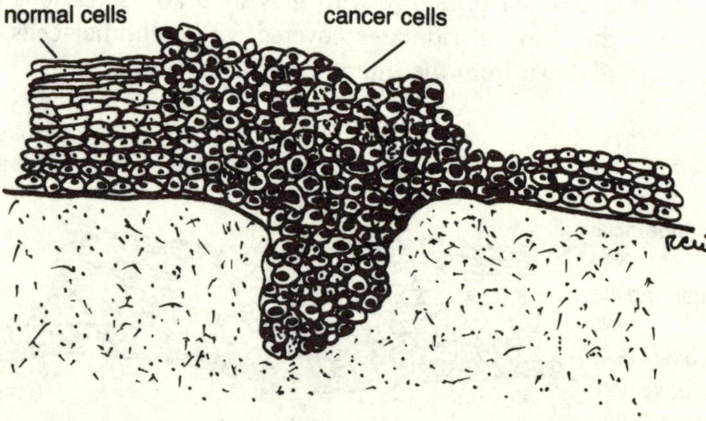

Squamous (epidermoid) cancer of the cervix. The cells at left show a normal, orderly development from young cells on the bottom to more mature cells on top. The cancerous cells at right are totally disarranged, and are pushing their way into the inner region of the cervix.

Several stages can be seen under the microscope as cells of the cervix undergo abnormal changes. Many words are used to describe the different changes (discussed fully under the biopsy section on page 42), but the terms usually refer to precancerous conditions that are 100 percent curable. Although specific cell changes can be seen microscopically in stages preceding cervical cancer and in early cervical cancer itself, there are usually no symptoms. The only way of detecting early cervical cancer is by the Pap test.

THE PAP TEST

The Pap test is a routine method of collecting cells from the cervix, having them analyzed, and then determining whether or not abnormal cell changes are taking place.

The Pap test is believed to have saved the lives of millions of women; the death rate from cervical cancer has declined by 70 percent in the forty years since the Pap test was introduced. All women should have the Pap test performed on a regular basis. The test is simple and painless and is the most sensitive and accurate screening test for detecting cervical cancer.

The Pap test is named for the Greek-American medical scientist George N. Papanicolaous. Working at Cornell Medical School in New York City in the early 1940s, Papanicolaous hoped to pinpoint the time of peak fertility in a women's ovulating cycle. Although he never did discover the critical index for fertility, he found that the growth patterns of cells could be evaluated if they were collected from the cervix on a glass slide. This technique, now simply called the Pap test, is still used today for detecting cervical cancer or cervical abnormalities.

For a Pap smear to be completely accurate, women should make certain that they are not inadvertently camouflaging the true condition of the cervical cells. Some physicians believe it is possible to alter the test results through douches, spray deodorants, or spermicidal jellies and creams. For a completely accurate Pap test, keep the following suggestions in mind.

• Never douche before your Pap test. Douching may clear away too many cells from the cervix.

• Consider postponing your appointment if you are just completing a menstrual period. Even if you are staining only slightly, it sometimes happens that too much blood will cloud the results of a Pap test, and you will have to have the test repeated.

• If possible, avoid vaginal sprays, foam, and other spermicidal creams that you might normally use for birth conrol for 72 hours before the test. (Your mate can use a condom.)

To take a Pap smear, the physician will spread the walls of the vagina with a speculum. Then another instrument—either a shaped wooden spatula similar to a tongue depressor, or a cotton-tipped swab—is inserted into the vagina to collect the cells to be studied.

After the cells are collected, they are placed on a slide. The slide is then "fixed," usually by being sprayed with a fixative solution, and sent to a laboratory where it is examined by a cytologist, a specialist in the microscopic study of the cells.

Self-Testing Pap Test Kits

Most Pap tests today are done in a physician's office. Some women's health groups, however, have advocated the use of self-testing kits, particularly for high-risk women who must have frequent tests. With a self-testing kit you can collect the cells from one's own cervix and then send them to a laboratory for processing. The self-testing kits have been suggested for two reasons: Women are given greater self-reliance in their own health care, and they save the cost of an office visit. There are several ways in which you can collect vaginal secretions. At present, none of the methods is 100 percent perfect. All involve far greater risk of error than if a physician collected the Pap smear. Until women can be given a device that safely and accurately collects cervical cells, we will not recommend or encourage self-testing Pap test kits.

In addition to the problem of collecting the cells, women must be extremely diligent in evaluating the laboratories where their Pap tests are being read. The most serious problem of the Pap test done at home, however, is that it eliminates a general office exam that also includes breast, pelvic, and rectal examinations. Since breast cancer is still the number-one cause of deaths from cancer in women, it is important that women receive regular check-ups. Can't a woman give herself a breast self-examination? Yes, she can, but studies show that many women today do not.

If the cost of office visits is a factor for you, rather than ignore a regular check-up, we encourage you to find a good hospital clinic or a women's health organization that offers medical services.

Laboratory Analysis of Pap Tests

One of the questions that most worries women after they receive the results of a Pap test is, "How do I know that the lab report was an accurate one? Since laboratories are subject to human error, mightn't they mix up my slide with someone else's or give me an inaccurate report?"

The answer is, of course, "Yes, laboratories do sometimes make mistakes." We learned recently of a young mother who eventually died of cervical cancer because of a laboratory report mix-up. In this particular case the physician told her she was fine!

It is crucial that you have not just a competent physician, but one who knows how to evaluate the laboratory that reads your Pap smears. In a well-run, well-managed laboratory, the pathologist will routinely review random slides designated as normal. This is a double-check on the initial screeners.

You might want to ask your physician why he or she chose the laboratory used—because of price, convenience, or quality. The correct answer should be obvious. To further protect yourself, you might also tell your physician that you would like to receive the laboratory report personally. After you have a Pap test, the usual procedure is to call back in a week or two for the results. Sometimes you receive a postcard that tells you the result. Ask your physician to send the results of the cytology report directly to you. This will keep your physician on his or her toes, protect you from a lost report, and give you the opportunity to be more aware of your own physical condition.

Will asking to have a report mailed to you add to the cost of your office visit? It shouldn't. For convenience, however, you might want to leave a self-addressed, stamped envelope with the nurse.

PAP SMEAR CLASSIFICATIONS

Although some physicians are now using only three major categories to define Pap smear classifications (benign, precancerous, and invasive cancer), this is an oversimplification. If your physician tells you that you have a "precancerous" condition, make certain you know exactly what he or she is talking about and what options for treatment exist.

The numerical system is the one most commonly used today, and it is the system we will use in this book. It is important to remember that on Pap test results *negative* always means that there are *no* abnormal cells present. *Positive* means that there *are* abnormal cells present.

Class 1 Negative for cancer cells
Class 2 Negative for atypical cells (usually suggesting infection or inflammation)
Class 3 Atypical doubtful (perhaps a mild dysplasia, perhaps worse)
Class 4 Suspicious for cancer cells (perhaps a severe dysplasia, a carcinoma *in situ*, or a real invasive cancer)
Class 5 Positive (cancer cells are seen; this might still be a very

severe dysplasia or carcinoma *in situ*, but cancer seems most likely.)

If Your Pap Test Result Is Class 1

A Class 1 Pap test result means that you have a completely normal smear with no sign whatsoever of any abnormal cells. Your physician undoubtedly will tell you to return in another year for your complete exam. Most physicians believe that you should have the Pap test done every year. Some clinics and some physicians, however, follow the 1980 controversial guidelines of the American Cancer Society, which suggests that if you have had negative Pap smears for two consecutive years and you are not a high-risk person, then you need not return for another test for three years. This guideline was developed on the basis of statistical studies that indicate that even if you have carcinoma *in situ*, it would take as many as five to thirty years to develop into invasive cancer. Many researchers and clinicians put that figure at ten years. Using ACS logic, if you went every three years for a Pap smear, it would still be possible to detect the disease in time for a near-perfect cure, and the cost of screening would be less.

The basic problem with the every-third-year Pap test is that it eliminates the rest of the office exam, which should be done each year, that is, the breast, pelvic, and rectal examinations. Still another problem is that in some rare instances, invasive cancer has been known to develop quickly and spread within a year. The women in these cases slip through the net of detection by waiting three years. An annual Pap test is also a safety valve—if your Pap test was misdiagnosed last year, this year's test probably will correct the error.

If Your Pap Test Result Is Class 2

Class 2 Pap test results usually indicate an easily curable inflammation or infection. If your Pap smear findings are usually

Class 1, don't worry. However, your physician will suggest that you return for a second test within a relatively short period of time, usually about three months. It is very important that you do so.

Will you be charged for a full office visit the second time if you only have a Pap test done? Discuss this with your physician. If the cost is too high, consider going to a clinic for a second test, but *do* inform your own physician of the results.

If after a second Pap smear you still have a Class 2 result, your physician will try to determine what problem exists and how to treat it. After you have been treated for the infection or inflammation, or after waiting at the suggestion of your physician to see whether the condition heals spontaneously, you should have the Pap smear repeated a third time. In most instances it will revert to a Class 1. If it does not, your physician might consider using some of the treatments described in the section on Class 3 Pap smear results (page 44).

If Your Pap Test Result Is Class 3

When your Pap smear is a Class 3, you have what generally is considered to be a precancerous condition. Class 3 means that the pathologist reading the Pap smear slide saw some abnormal cells or cell changes generally associated with dysplasia.

Dysplasia means an abnormal growth and/or development of cells. Although it is called a precancerous condition, it is important to remember that dysplasia may *never* develop into carcinoma *in situ* or invasive cancer, and that mild dysplasia is known to regress and heal spontaneously. Dysplasia affects only the surface layer of cells, and these cells do not invade the deeper tissues. (See the illustration of normal and dysplastic cells on page 34.) Many studies suggest, however, that these dysplastic changes are present before cervical cancer develops in women and so are a matter of concern.

How will your physician be able to distinguish a dysplastic

condition from a cancerous one? First, by the results of the Pap smear, which will be classified 3 or 4. Next you will be checked with a colposcope, and then you will have a biopsy. Frequently a colposcopic exam will give a very clear picture of cell changes on the cervix.

Colposcopy

The colposcopic exam is not done as routinely in the United States as it is in Europe, where it was originally developed. Women sometimes dislike this exam because they must lie on their backs with feet up on stirrups longer than for a Pap smear. The exam takes between five and twenty minutes and is painless. The colposcope itself looks like an odd pair of binoculars attached to a stand. The instrument never enters the body. It is a specially designed microscope used by the physician to see the tissues of the cervix.

If you are to be given a colposcopic exam, you will first have your vagina opened with a speculum in the usual way. After the cervix has been exposed, a special solution of acetic acid is applied to the vagina. Acetic acid is the same as white table vinegar. It may feel cold or sting. Then the physician will move the colposcope close to your vagina and look for an area of abnormal tissues. Because the colposcope magnifies the view, the physician will actually be able to see surface features that are known to represent dysplasia.

One thing to keep in mind regarding colposcopy is the proficiency of the colposcopist. Some physicians have been trained thoroughly through hospital projects. Any interested physician who has not been trained can take a weekend course in colposcopy and then purchase a colposcope for $1,500 to $10,000. Just because a physician owns a colposcope, however, does not necessarily mean that he or she is experienced in using it. Since the procedure is uncomfortable and can be time consuming, make certain you find an experienced colposcopist—someone who does the procedure a few times each day that he or she has office sessions. How will you find out that information? Ask.

Colposcopy exams are expensive; also be certain you ask about the cost in advance. The cost can range from $35 to $100. You might find out that a physician who does colposcopies once a week is charging much more than a physician who performs them routinely. On the other hand, the experienced colposcopist might be more than you can afford. Always try to go with experience. If you cannot afford a private colposcopic exam, ask your physician to direct you to the best available clinic.

If you are trying to find a good colposcopist on your own, call the chief of gynecology at your hospital and ask to whom he or she refers most colposcopy patients. Then ask, is it because that specialist is good, or because he or she is the only one in the area and you have no other choice?

After making your decision, use the same criteria with which you would judge any other physician. Feel confident that you are with a person you trust, or switch.

Biopsies

If after the colposcopy the physician is still in doubt about the condition of your cervix, most likely you will be given a small punch biopsy. A punch biopsy involves taking about 1⁄16 or 1⁄8 inch of skin from the affected area, usually from the side of the cervix, near the os (the cervical opening).

The procedure is practically painless because the nerves of the cervix are distributed rather sparsely. There is only one usual side effect—minor bleeding—which can be controlled with simple pressure or an astringent. On rare occasions you will need a stitch or two. Your physician might suggest you wait a few days before having sexual intercourse.

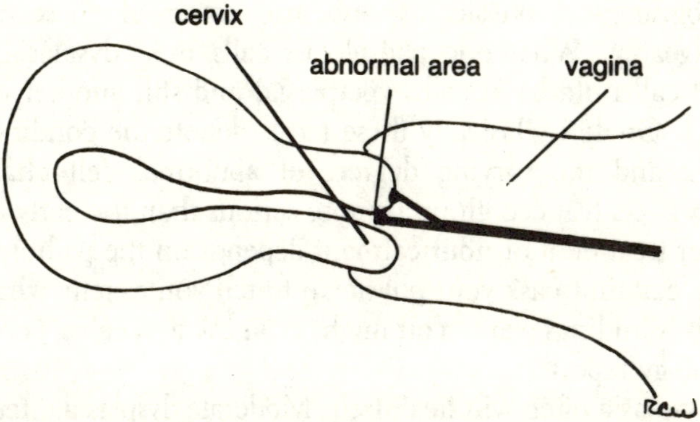

Punch biopsy of an abnormal area near the opening of the cervical canal.

The biopsy report will tell the physician in more detail about your condition. The language for classifying cervical biopsies is more complex than that used for Pap tests, and to complicate matters further, different laboratories sometimes use different terminology. The following are the terms most often used.

Mild dysplasia	Mild basal cell hyperplasia	Cervical intraepithelial neoplasia (CIN) Grade I
Moderate dysplasia	Moderate basal cell hyperplasia	CIN Grade II
Severe dysplasia, carcinoma *in situ*	Severe basal cell hyperplasia, atypical basal cell hyperplasia, carcinoma *in situ*	CIN Grade III

Pathologists and physicians also use some of these terms interchangeably. What one pathologist calls mild dysplasia, another will call mild basal cell hyperplasia, and still another might call it CIN Grade I. Basically these terms denote the condition of the cervix and the varying degrees of abnormal cell changes. Obviously the advanced group is more serious than the early ones. Since your treatment or nontreatment depends on the pathologist's report, be certain to ask your physician to tell you exactly what the pathologist's findings were. You might even ask to receive a copy of the pathology report.

Mild dysplasia often will heal itself. Moderate dysplasia often can be treated with cryosurgery (freezing) or cautery (burning). Severe dysplasia and/or carcinoma *in situ* usually is treated first with a conization, although some physicians today are still performing hysterectomies for this condition. Hysterectomies may, in some cases, be necessary. All three types of dysplasia have a virtually *perfect* cure rate.

Class 3 and 4 Pap Smears: The Gray Area

It is important to remember that disease patterns are not always so clear-cut that every pathologist reading a slide will make the same diagnosis. You might get a Class 3 *Pap* test result, indicating a mild dysplasia, even though the pathology report from the laboratory that studied your *biopsy* indicates a severe dysplasia, ordinarily associated with a Class 4 Pap smear.

Remember that the treatment you receive should not be based on a Pap smear, but on a *biopsy report*. It is your right to have a biopsy read by more than one pathologist, although this may be more expensive. If you are not satisfied with a biopsy report, talk it over with your physician. In most cases the treatment for mild or moderate dysplasia is the same, so deciding which you have may be academic. Just make certain you understand that with mild dysplasia you need not panic and rush into teatment. The

American Cancer Society reported on February 8, 1980, that "the best evidence is that most cases of dysplasia regress." Why not discuss this with your physician and give nature a chance to take its course? Do not, in any event, avoid your physician. If you have a biopsy that shows mild dysplasia, or if the diagnosis has been made from a colposcopic exam, and you and your physician have decided against any form of treatment, make certain to return for check-ups. You will want to know whether the condition has, in fact, regressed.

Treatment for Class 3 and Class 4 Conditions

If biopsy-proven mild dysplasia does not regress naturally, there are several forms of minimal treatment that can be given in a physician's office. *Cautery* is a technique for burning away the affected tissue with a simple electric heating unit, the hot cautery machine (electrocautery or thermo-cautery) or a more sophisticated laser unit. The cautery machine is a pen-shaped instrument with a tilted tip perhaps an inch long. It is hooked up to a small heating unit. After exposing the cervix with the speculum, the physician inserts the probe and burns away the abnormal cells. There is sometimes mild pain, but it lasts only a few seconds. Afterward you might have some heavy, usually bloody discharge for a week. You might feel some tenderness in the area. Generally within two weeks the area is healed. It is best not to have sexual intercourse for at least two to three weeks after cauterization. Some physicians suggest no sexual intercourse for as long as six weeks afterward.

Laser treatment is still being developed and is used at certain research centers. The laser machine looks like a large dentist's drill, but no part of it touches your body. Once you are positioned, the beam is aimed at the cervix and the tissue is destroyed. Time will tell whether the laser is better than the electrocautery now widely used.

Cryosurgery (or cryocautery) is a much newer technique for eliminating abnormal cells. If your physician does not have the machine for this treatment, you will be referred elsewhere. If your physician has a machine, the expense should be about the same as for a hot cautery. A cryosurgery unit looks like a large oxygen tank to which a type of handgun is attached. The gas in the tank is not oxygen, but carbon dioxide or nitrous oxide. The gun is fitted with a metal tip, in various sizes to fit the size of the cervix. When the metal tip touches the cervix, the gas is released, and within two minutes or so the area is frozen and the abnormal cells killed. You might feel the cold, and you might experience a sensation that is similar to menstrual cramp, but only briefly. As with the hot cautery, you may have a heavy watery discharge. This lasts for about a week, and you should avoid sexual intercourse for about two to six weeks. Recent critical review of experience with cryosurgery suggests that it may not be as effective as hot cautery.

For both types of treatments, you might be given vaginal creams that are supposed to help speed the healing process; not everyone agrees they do. Recurrence of dysplasia after any treament must be looked for.

Is there a specific time in your cycle that is best for cautery or cryosurgery? Yes. Right after a menstrual period is best for either.

Serious side effects from either procedure are unlikely. If you have had a pelvic inflammatory disease (PID) in the past, however, you are at higher risk. Pelvic inflammatory diseases are infections caused by anything from an intrauterine device (IUD) to a virus to gonorrhea or other bacteria. Usually PID affects the uterus, the fallopian tubes, and/or the ovaries.

If you have had PID, after cryosurgery or cautery you might have high fever, back pain, or possibly heavy clotting. Should this happen, call your doctor immediately. You will be given an antibiotic that should clear the problem up. While these side effects are not generally serious if treated effectively, they can be frightening.

Conization

It is possible that instead of cryosurgery or cautery your physician will suggest a conization—a type of cone-shaped biopsy used for both diagnostic and therapeutic purposes. Conizations usually are not performed more than once, because a greater amount of tissue is removed than with the tiny punch biopsy, which is used only for diagnostic purposes. Conization is a minimal treatment, but not all doctors agree that it is necessary in all cases of dysplasia. Remember that you should not permit any treatment without at least having a punch biopsy, particularly if conization is suggested. Usually conization is reserved for cases of severe dysplasia and carcinoma *in situ*. It is a specialized procedure that carries its own set of problems and risks (see pages 49–51 for a complete discussion of conization).

If your physician suggests conization for treatment of dysplasia, ask whether this is his or her usual recommendation or whether he or she feels it is the best treatment in your particular case. Be certain you understand fully the reasons for a suggested conization, and be certain that *you* are satisfied that the lesser treatments would not be better for you. If you are not totally satisfied with your physician's explanation, get a second opinion. Your insurance coverage may even include the cost of a second opinion, since conization requires a hospital stay.

Silver Nitrate

In the past, some women were treated for dysplasia with silver nitrate sticks. This is an obsolete treatment and it should no longer be used, since the nitrate does not effectively destroy the abnormal cells. This is a good treatment to *refuse* if it is ever offered to you.

If Your Pap Test Result Is Class 4

The Class 4 Pap smear frequently reflects carcinoma *in situ;* however, it can also indicate a less serious condition such as mild dysplasia. Carcinoma *in situ* will be diagnosed in about 45,000 women in 1981. The cure rate in these women is virtually 100 percent.

Cells normally change in a predictable manner. With carcinoma *in situ*, however, the changes as cells grow to maturity are abnormal. Individual cells are less similar to each other. Instead of new cells growing to maturity, a microscope will show more cells dividing, which indicates a rapid cell formation as occurs with cancer. Some physicians call carcinoma *in situ* a true precursor to cancer.

If your Pap test result is a Class 4, you will be given a colposcopic exam and a punch biopsy. The results of the punch biopsy will help your physician determine what treatment is best for you. If you have requested the pathologist's report for yourself, you might find that while your physician told you he or she suspected carcinoma *in situ*, the report reads severe dysplasia or CIN Grade III. Keep in mind that within medical circles one doctor's severe dysplasia is another doctor's carcinoma *in situ*. Even with today's sophisticated diagnostic equipment, the varying degrees of dysplasia and carcinoma *in situ* are debated. Don't be concerned about the academic argument. If you have either of these conditions, your treatment choices will probably be the same: conization or hysterectomy.

Making a treatment choice is very important to you. Conization is a minimal procedure. If you have never had children, conization may or may not interfere with your ability to conceive and deliver a baby. Hysterectomies, on the other hand, leave you sterile. Always.

If you feel you want minimal treatment, don't be talked out of it without a second opinion. Don't be intimidated if your doctor verbally agrees with your choice for conization while giving the silent impression that you have made the wrong decision.

You may even make the choice of having *no treatment*. Although carcinoma *in situ* is the earliest form of cancer, cases of it have been known to regress without any treatment. In a statement of February 26, 1980, regarding the frequency of Pap tests, the American Cancer Society said: "Our concern involving the Pap test comes from treating cases of dysplasia and CIS (cancer *in situ)* that might have regressed spontaneously. We do not know precisely how often this occurs, or how long it takes for a case to regress, but the best evidence is that most cases of dysplasia regress, and that while the proportions of CIS that regress are unknown, any regressions that do occur, either naturally or because they were originally misread, do so within a year of diagnosis." Physicians today generally suggest you accept treatment since carcinoma *in situ* does not frequently regress.

Conization

The side effects of conization or cone biopsy can be more serious than those of an average punch biopsy, and so this procedure is always done in a hospital. What might happen first, however, is that your physician will do an endocervical curettage. This is a scraping of the cervical canal sometimes also performed after conization. It is done to collect tissue for microscopic evaluation from higher up in the endocervical region than the area from which cells are taken in a conization.

For a conization, you will first be admitted to the hospital, then your physician may order some routine tests. When conization does take place, it is usually done under general anesthesia. Local anesthesia might in some way obscure the area of the cervix from which the physician wishes to collect the cells.

For a discussion of preoperative tests and questions to ask anesthesiologists, see Chapter 11.

The conization procedure serves a twofold purpose: diagnostic and therapeutic. The cone shape of the section removed (like an inverted pyramid) is designed to capture all the abnormal cells. This procedure removes the abnormal cells that are no longer on the external surface but are spreading up into the cervical canal.

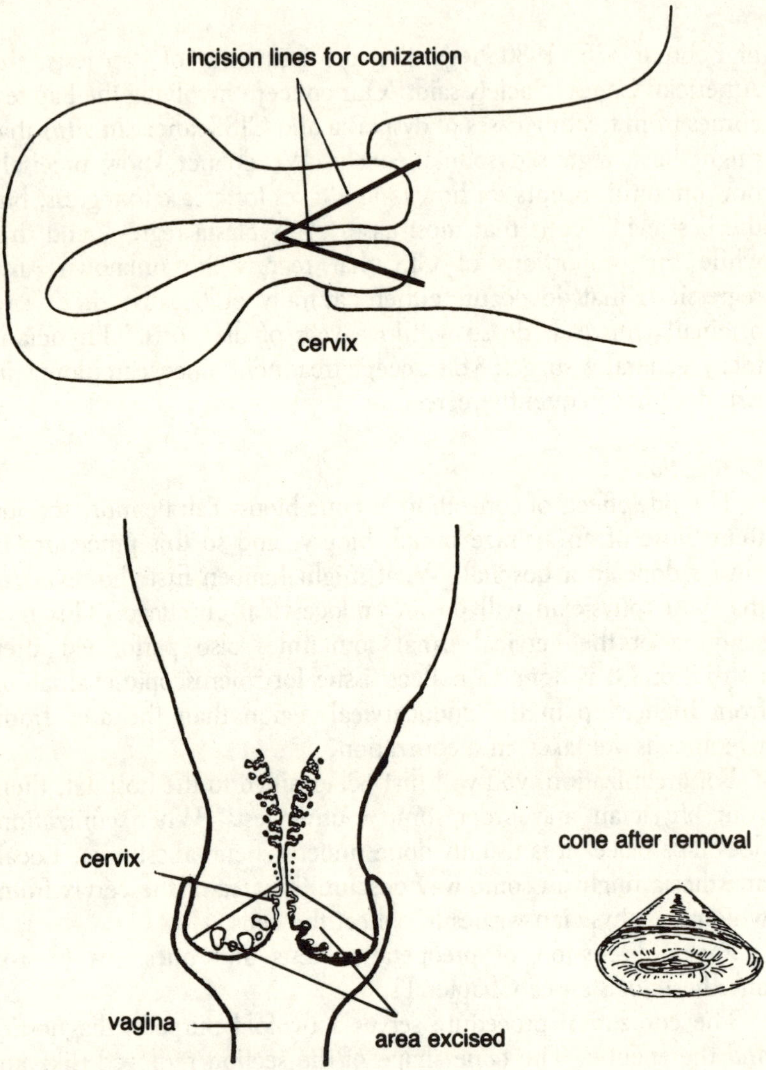

The cone biopsy of the cervix (conization). The removal of a cone-shaped section ensures that all abnormal cells will be removed.

The cone will extend to a point where normal cells should be seen. From a therapeutic point of view, conization is the treatment for carcinoma *in situ*.

After the cone-shaped section of the cervix is removed, your physician will send the tissue to a pathologist, who will make a dozen or more different slides and then determine whether or not any additional abnormal cells escaped the treatment. In this way conization is also a diagnostic procedure.

Immediate side effects of conization include bleeding and the possibility of infection. The bleeding may last for several weeks, and you will not be able to have sexual intercourse for about six weeks.

A long-range side effect is that your physician may have difficulty detecting any future abnormalities of the cervix because its shape may change during healing. Conization may scar the cervix and in some instances either interfere with ability to conceive or possibly cause the cervix to open up early in pregnancy. This results in miscarriages or premature deliveries. Just make certain that if you change physicians after having conization and later become pregnant, you have an obstetrician who watches your condition carefully. If the scar on the cervix interferes with cervical dilation at the time of labor and delivery, you might have to have a cesarean delivery. Despite all the side effects, remember: If you want a child, and you have early cancer, conization can offer you the chance to conceive and have a child or even have several children, whereas a hysterectomy always leaves you sterile.

Hysterectomy

If after conization the carcinoma *in situ* returns, even once, some physicians today will suggest either a conventional hysterectomy or a modified radical hysterectomy. Hysterectomies are a more definitive treatment, since you will never have to worry about ever having carcinoma *in situ* of the cervix again. If the thought of cancer scares you, if you can't live with the notion that some of these early cancer cells may be hiding in the uterus and that you are still harboring the disease, then a hysterectomy will give you peace of mind. Don't make the decision quickly or without a second opinion from a highly qualified gynecologic oncologist.

Physicians are most likely to suggest a hysterectomy for women who are past childbearing age. But some women in their fifties make the choice to keep all their reproductive organs, even women who never wanted to have children.

Some physicians suggest immediate surgery for carcinoma *in situ*. Again, get a second opinion. If you decide on the surgery, be certain you understand what type of hysterectomy is planned.

The conventional hysterectomy involves removal of the cervix and the uterus and nothing more. The modified radical hysterectomy involves removal of the upper part of the vagina—that area where the cervix is attached—as well as the cervix and uterus. This is a riskier procedure because of the greater dissection of pelvic tissue involved. This bigger operation is used when the abnormal cells have been found near the end of the cervix or even on the upper vagina. If this procedure is suggested, make certain you are with a specially trained gynecologic surgery team.

If you and your physician agree that a hysterectomy is the best treatment, ask to be told of all planned tests and also to be introduced to the anesthesiologist as discussed in Chapter 11 on treatment. A hysterectomy generally requires a seven- to ten-day hospital stay.

How will you feel emotionally? Since the cure rate is about 100 percent, you'll probably feel pretty good, at least initially. Will you later have other emotional side effects? Perhaps. Read the section on page 57 where we discuss this in greater depth.

If Your Pap Test Result Is a Class 5

Although a Class 5 Pap smear usually means invasive cancer, it is also possible that after the biopsy report you will be found to have only carcinoma *in situ*. Still another possibility is a microinvasive cancer of the cervix, which is the earliest form of invasive cancer. In this case the tumor intrudes only a few millimeters into the part of the cervix that contains the blood vessels, the connective tissue, and the nerves.

If you are ever diagnosed as having microinvasive cancer, the question of treatment is crucial and there is no consensus as to the best approach. Some physicians feel it should not be treated in the same way as invasive cancer of the cervix; other physicians disagree. What should you do? Find a team of surgeons and pathologists who have had experience treating this type of cancer, and then go with the decision that feels best to you. Consult the doctor within you. Weigh the risks and benefits, and then decide.

Sometimes, however, you might have invasive cancer and the Pap smear report will be negative. This happens extremely rarely and no one really knows why. For some reason, the cancer may not shed cells, or the abnormal cells may be masked by blood and infection. Your physician usually will be able to detect invasive cancer of the cervix just by feeling or seeing the cervix. Also, you might be given a colposcopic exam and a biopsy as well. If you have invasive cancer, it is unlikely that it will go unnoticed by a trained physician.

With invasive cervical cancer, cells have formed a mass or tumor, which is a collection of abnormal cells, and some of these cells have shot off from the site and invaded the surrounding tissue. Once these cells get into the blood stream or the lymph nodes, they are carried to different organs. With cervical cancer, the other organs affected usually include the immediate surrounding ones, that is, the deep pelvic tissues. Eventually, if left unchecked, the cancer spreads to the lungs or blocks the kidneys, this is fatal.

Even with invasive cervical cancer, particularly in the earliest stage, the chance for cure is very good, as the story of Cholee indicates.

Cholee was just twenty when she left her Montana reservation to marry an FBI agent. She had three children in six years and said she couldn't count how many times they had moved. Because of her children, household chores, and moves, Cholee never had a doctor who regularly took care of her.

At Cholee's first full gynecological exam in years, she was found to have an abnormal Pap smear, and a cone biopsy showed that she had an early invasive cancer of the cervix.

In her case, radical hysterectomy was suggested. The surgery was performed when she was twenty-eight. She left the hospital two weeks later feeling fine—even "well rested," she said.

Cholee kept in close contact with the physician who treated her, despite continued moves because of her husband's job. She finally settled in an area within one hour of the hospital where she was originally treated and returns faithfully to her physician for her yearly check-ups. Fifteen years have passed and she has had no recurrence of disease.

Treatment for early invasive cancer of the cervix is usually surgery in younger, otherwise healthy women. Most often it is a radical hysterectomy involving removal of the cervix, the upper part of the vagina, the body of the uterus, adjacent deep pelvic tissue and lymph nodes (it is through the lymph nodes that cervical cancer spreads). The ovaries and fallopian tubes also are usually, but not necessarily, removed.

The surgery may rarely be followed by radiation treatments.

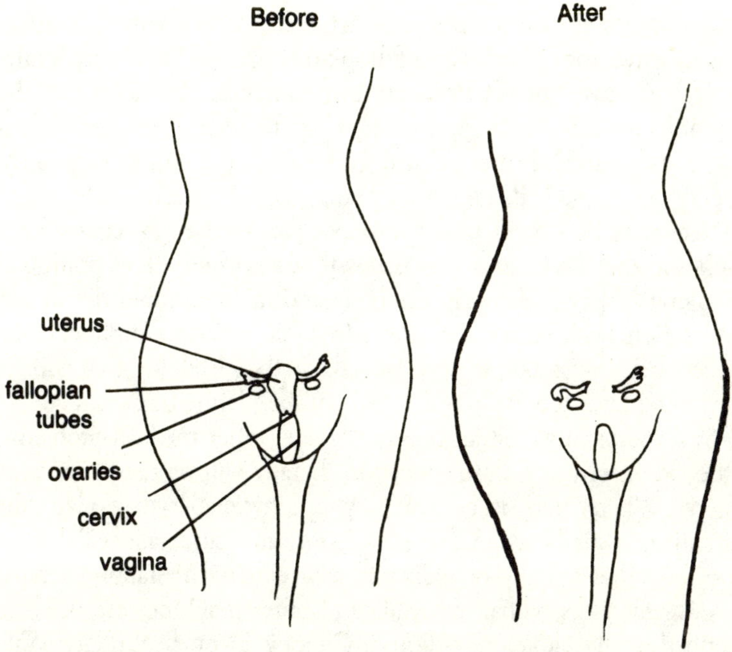

Hysterectomy. The figure at left shows the position of the organs. In the figure at right, the uterus and cervix have been removed. In this case, the fallopian tubes and ovaries have been left intact. Often, they are also removed.

Chemotherapy also is being used on an experimental basis in addition to surgery at a few major teaching centers.

Ask your physician to explain anything about the surgical procedure that doesn't seem clear to you. Don't accept "don't worry about a thing" for an answer. In fact, if prior to surgery you feel that the doctor is not giving you adequate time to discuss treatment, pin him down. Physicians trained and experienced in treating this cancer are busy, but should be able to explain all the aspects of your case.

Your major concern should be whether or not your physician plans to leave your ovaries and fallopian tubes in. This is especially true if you have not yet undergone menopause. By depriving the body of its source of estrogen, removal of the ovaries creates what is known as "surgical menopause." Because the surgical change happens so quickly, its effects can be especially severe.

There may be cancer near the upper part of the vagina, where it attaches to the cervix, and if so this will be removed. (This portion of the vagina is very high up in the body and its loss should not in any way interfere with sexual activities.) In some very rare instances, the bladder and lower bowel also are taken; the need for this will be determined by extensive biopsies and will be planned in advance.

For some patients, either because of age, other medical problems, or the extent of the disease, radiation therapy will be used instead of surgery. When there is a choice, your physician will explain the alternatives; usually when a choice exists, the cure rate will be the same for either surgery or radiation. For external radiation therapy, linear accelerators, cobalt 60 units and other machines are used, as described in the radiation section of Chapter 11 on treatments. With tiny internal radioactive sources, radiation can be placed directly in the body. This is called *intracavity placement*, and it is usually done under general anesthesia. The radiation sources might be as large as a pen or as slender as the lead in a pencil. In the case of cancer of the cervix, radioactive sources will be placed in the cervix and vagina close to the parametrium—the tissue next to the cervix and upper vagina—where the tumor is known to spread.

The radioactive sources often are inserted in two steps. First a carrier for the radioactive material—usually radium, cesium or cobalt—is placed inside. After its position has been checked by x-ray and the patient has returned to her room, a special applicator is used to place the radioactive source into the carrier. This after-loading technique is almost universally available at modern hospitals.

Chemotherapy and immunotherapy have also been used with varied results. The use of chemotherapeutic agents either in initial treatment or for treatment of recurrence of cancer of the cervix has achieved neither great popularity nor great success. (Experimental use of chemotherapy is underway at major teaching centers and has occasionally yielded improvement or sustained remission in a small number of cases.)

Immunotherapy, the manipulation of the immune mechanisms of the body, has also been tried, but it has not produced any substantially good results for treatment of cervical cancer.

EMOTIONAL SIDE EFFECTS

While recovery from any form of surgery can be physically difficult, there can be emotional side effects as well.

Depression is perhaps the most common side effect. Women actually do suffer a form of grief when they lose a part of their body, even an organ with a disease that may have killed them. Young women who lose their reproductive potential have still another problem to cope with—not only have they lost a part of themselves, but they have forever lost their ability to conceive and bear a child.

Robin was just twenty-one when she learned she had an early cervical cancer, and she was treated by a radical hysterectomy. Although she admitted she was angry about the surgery, she had a good rapport with her physician and was pleasant during her entire hospital stay.

At her three-month check-up, Robin was apparently overwhelmed with grief. The physician suggested that it was quite normal to have such feelings after major surgery and that some women found it helpful to see a psychotherapist.

Robin became furious at his suggestion. "I am *not* crazy, but I am depressed. My problem is not emotional; it is physical. Before surgery my boyfriend and I had a terrific sex life; now I feel nothing. What happened, I'm sure, is that in the course of the surgery my nerve cells were shifted. There is no feeling of pleasure anymore. Not only will I never be able to enjoy children, but I will never again be able to enjoy sex."

When it became clear that she would not seek psychiatric counseling, the physician spent a bit more time with her, explaining that there was no physical reason for her not to enjoy sex.

Six months later, Robin's sexual problems were over. She never sought therapy, but she was fortunate enough to have a few close friends who allowed her to grieve, comforted her when she mourned, and then gently told her that it was time to grow up. And she did, by using some wellsprings of inner strength that even she did not know existed. Usually, however, psychiatric help is most valuable.

Emotional side effects are not to be taken lightly. We can only urge women who are deeply depressed over surgery to get professional counseling. If you have good close friends to help you, all the better. Don't make emotional recovery difficult on yourself. This is a legitimate time to ask to see the liaison psychiatrist many hospitals use today. If your hospital doesn't have one, ask your physician to recommend a psychiatrist or other therapist.

Some physicians say, "Ask me, I'll help." Graciously accept the offer, but ask for professional help with your emotions if you think you need it. After all, you wouldn't ask your hairdresser for a manicure. Don't expect that a surgeon can necessarily do the job of a counselor. Many hospitals are incorporating special "cope" groups to help women adjust to the aftermath of surgery for cancer. Inquire about these at your hospital.

HOW CAN CERVICAL CANCER BE PREVENTED?

With today's detection methods, cancer of the cervix ought to be eliminated in our lifetime. Because the precancerous conditions are 100 percent curable and because the earliest stage of cancer, carcinoma *in situ,* has a virtually perfect cure rate, there is little reason for any woman today to lose her life to this disease.

How do you prevent cervical cancer? Since there is no certainty as to its cause, it is difficult to talk in terms of prevention. What you can do, however, is have Pap tests regularly. The big question today is what constitutes "regularly." For women who are promiscuous, regular might be every month. For other high-risk women, regular may be every six months. For the average woman, it is usually once a year. You should discuss this with your physician and decide how often is "regularly" for you.

Some women feel that the yearly test gives them peace of mind. Taking into account the human error factor, the yearly test is a safety valve. If your test last year was misread or misdiagnosed, this year is your double-check.

Despite the academic arguments among physicians regarding testing, do what you feel is best. Do not become disillusioned with the whole profession and say, "No one knows what they're talking about anymore." This is a self-defeating attitude. Do not be concerned with medical group in-fighting. Be concerned with yourself and your health. Find a way to get regular check-ups. Do not compromise the only body you have.

RECOMMENDED ARTICLES

Brenner DE. Carcinoma of the cervix—a review. *American Journal of Medical Science* 284:31–48.

Chapter Four

The DES-Cancer Connection

Before reading about the dangers of the synthetic hormone DES, Nancy liked to compare her own easy pregnancies with the difficult pregnancies her mother had endured. She used the same obstetrician to deliver her children that her mother had used when Nancy herself was born. This fatherly figure frequently reminded Nancy, "You are a very lucky young lady to have such an easy time carrying children. When your mother was pregnant with you, she spent most of her time in bed."

Because the physician feared that Nancy's mother might have a miscarriage, he not only suggested she stay in bed for most of her pregnancy, but he also gave her vitamin shots and a hefty supply of hormone pills. The physician told Nancy's mother that the pills were a wonder drug that would keep her hormones "in balance" and prevent a miscarriage. Nancy was born a plump, healthy child, and Nancy's mother was very grateful to the physician who helped her.

After Nancy had her third child she began to experience a heavy mucus discharge. While at the physician's office one day she began to read about DES. She later said, "I read the story and shook my head in disbelief that such a thing could happen to women."

A few days later as she was thinking about the DES story, Nancy panicked. "I remembered that somewhere in the story the writer referred to hormone pills that sounded like the hormones my mother took. I thought of all those young women who might be affected by cancer, and I realized that I could be one of those women."

Nancy calmed herself; she phoned her physician to ask about DES. The nurse who took the call said, "Don't worry about it; just come in for your regular Pap smears and you will be fine."

The fact is, Pap smears may *not* detect the type of cancer associated with DES. Office exams for DES-exposed daughters should also include colposcopies and biopsies. Being a persistent young woman, Nancy insisted that she speak with the physician about her worries concerning DES exposure. The physician had her return for a visit that included a colposcopic exam. Nancy was found to have a noncancerous condition related to DES, but a condition for which she will have to be watched carefully for the rest of her life.

WHAT IS DES?

The Department of Health, Education, and Welfare has a new public information campaign that calls DES "the wonder drug that women should wonder about." DES, technically called diethylstilbestrol, was marketed under many different brand names. All these brands are the same synthetic substances with properties resembling estrogen, a female hormone. DES was considered a wonder drug in the 1940s because physicians believed the drug was preventing miscarriages by stopping the bleeding in early pregnancy that was associated with the tendency to miscarry.

As early as the 1920s and 1930s physicians realized that some uterine bleeding was related to estrogen withdrawal. If they gave women hormone injections, the bleeding stopped. In 1938, when British scientist E. C. Dobbs developed DES, it was a major medical breakthrough. Pills are not only less expensive than injections, but they can be easily prescribed. Physicians who suspected that women who bled in pregnancy might miscarry could now prescribe a wonder drug—the DES pill. Today physicians know that bleeding in early pregnancy is a common occurrence and does not necessarily mean a miscarriage will ensue. In the 1940s, however, physicians believed that if the pregnancy was to continue, the bleeding had to be stopped, and DES was now available to "protect" pregnancies.

The medical literature shows that it was two physicians in the Northeast who were chiefly responsible for the widespread acceptance of DES. They gave it to women who bled in pregnancy. The bleeding stopped. The women had what appeared to be normal children. DES seemed to work. As it later turned out, however, the physicians' conclusions were based on incomplete research and inconclusive evidence. No comparative studies were done, and no drug agency existed at the time to monitor new prescription drugs.

It was at least ten years before researchers began to seriously question the usefulness of DES. In a controlled comparative study of DES at the University of Chicago, physicians prescribed DES to one group of women and a placebo, a pill of no medical value, to others. When the results were compared, the data indicated that DES as a means of protecting pregnancies was of doubtful value.

The Chicago study initiated a debate in medical circles that would go on for almost twenty years during which doctors continued to prescribe the pill. As late as 1962 the National Academy of Science and the National Research Council rated DES as "possibly effective" in preventing miscarriages. And women continued taking the drug.

During this entire period, no one noticed any adverse side effects of DES. It wasn't until the late 1960s that two physicians at

Massachusetts General Hospital in Boston, Dr. Arthur L. Herbst, a gynecologist, and Dr. Robert Scully, a pathologist, were able to pinpoint the hazards of DES.

In the course of their work these doctors began to see cases in which young women had a peculiar type of vaginal cancer. Vaginal cancer is extremely rare and is generally detected only in women over sixty-five. In a single year, these physicians saw six or seven cases of a vaginal cancer with an unusual microscopic picture. These cases were more than they had seen in the preceding ten years. The form of cancer they observed is now known to be related almost exclusively to patients with DES exposure.

An epidemiological investigation ensued: What factors in the backgrounds of the young women might have been associated with this unusual type of cancer? Researchers considered cigarette smoking, pregnancies, sexual activity, and drug exposure. In the final analysis, most women shared a common factor—their mothers had received DES in the first three months of pregnancy. With the vast body of information available about DES, the way in which the genital tract responds to certain estrogens, and superb insight on the part of the investigators, an association between DES and cancer was established.

Due to the worldwide attention given to the studies, the practice of routinely giving the drug to pregnant women ended. In 1971 the Food and Drug Administration ordered a label to be placed on prescription for the drug warning pregnant women of its potential hazards.

EFFECTS OF DES

The most serious side effect in DES-exposed daughters has been a type of cancer called clear-cell adenocarcinoma. The cancer gets its name because it arises in a gland: adenocarcinoma stands for cancer of the glandular epithelium. In the microscopic picture of the disease, clear spaces can be seen within the cells. It is believed that one in every 2,000 women whose mothers took the drug will be affected. Statistics are difficult to come by, however; some estimates suggest only one in 7,000, and others suggest one in 700. To date, scores of women in the United States have died as a result of cancer associated with DES. Worldwide, about 400 cases of human cancer related to DES have been reported. It has been estimated that between 4 and 6 million persons primarily in the United States have been affected by DES, if you include in that figure mothers who took the drug, their daughters, and their sons. (DES-exposed sons are also affected; some with minor genital problems, others with suspected sterility.)

Statistically, only a very small percentage of women will have DES-associated cancer, but if you or your daughter is one of those statistics, it is of little comfort to hear that most women will not develop serious side effects from the drug. The trauma experienced by women affected cannot be minimized by numbers.

In addition to the increased risk of cancer, women who were exposed to DES are affected by related conditions and problems, including vaginal and cervical adenosis, vaginal and uterine malformations, and vaginal hoods. These conditions are discussed at length beginning on page 000. Most of the related conditions are nonmalignant. Vaginal and cervical adenosis, however, may be associated with cancer.

DETECTING DES-RELATED CONDITIONS

If your mother took DES, or if you think she might have taken DES, you should decide immediately to become your own investigative reporter. Keep in mind that it was the DES administered during the first eighteen weeks of pregnancy that is now considered to have been the most harmful. Some researchers, however, have narrowed the time span, feeling that the period from eight to eighteen weeks is the most crucial.

Make every effort to contact the physician who cared for your mother during her pregnancy. Ask to see all the records that pertain to her pregnancy with you. If you cannot get any information and suspect that you have been exposed to DES, call a gynecologist experienced with DES cases and ask for an appointment for a complete check-up.

Some women have already been contacted by a physician, because on October 7, 1978, a Physician's Advisory from the Surgeon General of the United States was issued and mailed to all 400,000 physicians in the nation. They were urged to check their records carefully, even if it required searching through records twenty years old or more, in order to identify those female patients given DES.

It was suggested that physicians—

• notify women to whom they had prescribed the drug and advise them about the need for follow-up medical care for themselves or their children, sons as well as daughters.

• check their medical records carefully when approached by patients inquiring about possible past exposure to DES in order to provide these patients with information as accurate and complete as possible.

• provide this information to women *without charge.*

This is a monumental task, especially given our mobile society. No DES-exposed woman can necessarily count on being told about the possible risk she faces, so it is up to *you.* If you have been exposed to DES, finding out the facts might save your life.

It is crucial for you to find a physician who understands this disease. While many of the cases reported were in the Northeast, just because you live in the Mideast does not necessarily mean your mother was not given the drug. If you live in a small town, however, and know or think you were exposed, you may have to make a trip to the nearest major cancer center or university hospital to find a physician who can treat you or give you the basic tests to determine whether you have any DES-related cancer or other conditions.

If you do not know of a physician and wish a referral, contact a DES Action group. The addresses are listed in the appendix. You may call information for the telephone number of a DES Action group in your area.

If you are trying to determine whether or not you received DES, you should be aware of the names of the following drugs, all of which are DES substances.

Nonsteroidal estrogens

Benzestrol
Chlorotrianisene
Comestrol
Cyren A
Cyren B
Delvinal
DES
DesPlex
Diestryl
Dibestil
Dienestrol
Dienoestrol
Diethylstilbestrol Dipalmitate
Diethylstilbestrol Diphosphate
Diethylstilbestrol Dipropionate
Diethystilbenediol
Digestil
Domestrol
Estilben
Estrobene
Estrobene DP
Estrosyn
Fonatol
Gynben
Gyneben
Hexestrol
Hexoestrol
Hi-Bestrol
Menocrin
Meprane
Mestibol
Methallenestril
Microest
Mikarol
Mikarol forti
Milestrol
Monomestrol
Neo-Oestranol I
Neo-Oestranol II

Nonsteroidal estrogen-androgen combinations

Amperone
Di-Erone
Estan
Metystil
Teserene
Tylandril
Tylosterone

Nonsteroidal estrogen-progesterone combination

Progravidium

Vaginal cream—and suppositories with nonsteroidal estrogens

AVC cream with Dienestrol
Dienestrol cream

Nulabort
Oestrogenine
Oestromenin
Oestromon
Orestol
Pabestrol D
Palestrol
Restrol
Stil-Rol
Stilbal
Stilbestrol
Stilbestronate
Stilbetin
Stilbinol
Stilboestroform
Stilboestrol
Stilboestrol DP
Stilestrate
Stilpalmitate
Stilphostrol
Stilronate
Stilrone
Stils
Synestrin
Synestrol
Synthoestrin
Tace
Vallestril
Willestrol

EXAMINATIONS FOR DES CONDITIONS

If you think you were exposed to DES, make an appointment to see a physician. After talking with the physician and giving him or her a complete medical history, specify that you want the results of all tests even if cancer is not detected. Since uterine malformations may make conception or childbirth difficult, it is important that you be told of these conditions as well. The doctor should perform the following examinations.

• *Pelvic exam*. This is given to all women as a matter of routine. The physician will feel the cervix and uterus for any abnormalities. If you have a daughter, she should be examined as soon as she begins to menstruate. Some physicians prefer to examine DES-exposed daughters even earlier.

• *Pap smears*. Two types of Pap smears are performed for DES daughters, one with cells from the cervix and one with cells from the vagina.

• *Colposcopy*. This is an exam in which a microscope-like

instrument is used to look at the cervix. (A full discussion of colposcopy begins on page 41.) It is often included in the first visit of a DES daughter to a physician and then repeated only if abnormal Pap smears continue. Some physicians, however, feel the DES daughter should have repeated colposcopy for a lifetime.

• *Biopsy.* If the physician is in doubt about the findings of the other tests, you will be given a biopsy, which is simply the removal of a small bit of tissue to be examined under a microscope. This can usually be done right in the physician's office. (For a more complete discussion of the punch biopsy, see page 42.) After the exam you will be given a clean bill of health, told of a related condition, or told you may have cancer.

If you are told there is no sign of cancer after the first visit, can you rest peacefully? Maybe. It may mean that you are never going to develop cancer associated with DES, or it may mean that you are going to develop cancer but it simply has not happened yet. However, almost all cancers are detected at the first visit. There have been only five cases of DES-associated cancer reported after the first check-up was normal. It is highly likely that once you have had a check-up that is negative you need not worry.

CERVICAL AND VAGINAL ADENOSIS

In cervical and vaginal adenosis, collections of mucus-secreting cells become trapped under the lining of the vagina. If these particular cells are in the cervical canal, all is normal. But in the vagina and on the outside of the cervix they are out of place.

Because the mucus-secreting cells are usually trapped under the lining of the vagina and cannot be seen by the naked eye (a physician detects this using a colposcope), you probably will have no symptoms.

Although the abnormal distribution of mucus-secreting cells related to DES changes might be expected to cause mucus discharge, this rarely, if ever, happens. If you have a mucusy vaginal discharge, it is probably related to a common, treatable, "garden variety" vaginal condition and not at all related to adenosis.

What, then, *is* the treatment for adenosis? There is no need for treatment if you have adenosis. Some books and some physicians suggest that hot cautery or freezing might be useful. These are not effective in reversing DES-induced changes. If you have a mucus discharge, make certain that your physician determines its cause. Even if there is a mucus discharge for some other reason, consider letting the condition heal naturally within a few weeks before consenting to hot cautery or freezing.

Cervical adenosis can have other causes than DES exposure. Many years ago it was described in the German medical literature, and in the early 1940s it was named by Dr. A. Plaut, a pathologist at New York City's Beth Israel Hospital, when he described a similar case prior to the widespread use of DES. It is not, however, very commonly seen.

While adenosis is not proved to be a precursor to cancer, physicians who treat the cancer associated with DES usually find that women with cancer also have adenosis. Thus every case of adenosis might not turn into cancer, but almost every case of DES cancer does have an association with adenosis. Proof of any direct link between the two is lacking. In 1973 an epidemiological study indicated that women with adenosis were at high risk to develop conventional cervical cancer precursors. A more recent study in Boston by pathologist Stanley Robboy, however, suggested that there is *no* increased risk. If you have adenosis, nonetheless, be watched carefully.

If you have cervical or vaginal adenosis, you should have a check-up every six months to one year, probably for your lifetime. Included in that check-up may be the colposcopic exam. The costs of colposcopy can be high. Who pays the bill? Should you have to pay these fees for the rest of your life?

The DES Task Force has recommended that major insurance carriers cover the cost of physicians' fees. It recommends that studies be made of other sources for reimbursement, especially for women not covered by insurance plans. In addition, it recommends that women in college be given the service as part of their college health plan. In the event that National Health Insurance is adopted in the United States, the task force urged that DES coverage be included. If you have difficulty with payment now, contact a consumer group or your DES Action Group to see how you might be helped, or find a well-staffed clinic at a teaching hospital.

OTHER DES-RELATED CONDITIONS

Other conditions related to DES, but not associated with cancer, include vaginal and uterine malformations and vaginal hoods. Vaginal and uterine malformations include transverse ridges of the cervix and vagina and the T-shaped uterus. Transverse ridges are like tiny folds that run from side to side along the anterior wall of the vagina up toward the cervix.

The T-shaped uterus has been found in some women exposed to DES *in utero* (before birth). The shape of the cavity of the uterus is like a T rather than its usual pear shape. The uterus is smaller in size, and some women with this condition have problems with pregnancy and conception.

This connection was determined by Dr. Raymond Kaufman, who was at Beth Israel Medical Center in New York City before heading the staff at Baylor Institute in Texas. Previously DES was thought to affect only the cervix and vagina, but Dr. Kaufman determined that DES might also affect the upper part of the genital tract, which is the body of the uterus. As a result, Dr. Arthur L. Herbst, one of the original reporters of the link between DES and cancer, wrote in the *Journal of Reproductive Medicine* in 1979 on a study of pregnancies of 226 DES-exposed and 203 unexposed women. Herbst found that DES-exposed women had more frequent pregnancy losses and more problems with reproduction than did unexposed women. This association with DES, however, is still being debated.

What then should you do? Ask your physician to monitor you very closely during the time you are carrying a child.

DES-RELATED CANCER

If after your colposcopy and biopsy your physician says you have tissue changes associated with cancer, you can do one of two things. You can ask for a second pathology report; that is, ask for another pathologist's opinion. Or you can ask to see a second gynecologic oncologist to confirm the findings. The cost of a second opinion for major surgery is covered by insurance in most states. Ask the physicians how many cases of DES cancer he or she has seen and treated. If the answer is none, you will probably want to go elsewhere. If the answer is five, you may be in good hands, since there have been only about 400 cases worldwide.

DES-related cancer is amenable to treatment. For example, Janice was twenty-five years old when she learned she had vaginal cancer associated with DES. As a single parent with two young children, she was more than ordinarily concerned about her health. It was after a routine postpartum check-up that she was told she had an abnormal Pap smear. Janice had a second Pap test, and when that too was abnormal, she had a colposcopic exam and a biopsy. The tests revealed an early stage of cancer.

Janice had surgery four years ago and today considers herself cured, and doctors say her prognosis is excellent. Although many young women have emotional side effects from this type of surgery, Janice is happy to be alive. "I'm thinking more about my children than myself, I guess. My first worry was, who would take care of them? I never had the time to feel depressed about the surgery or this whole DES mess."

Cindy Lou, on the other hand, couldn't admit to herself that she might have cancer. In fact, Cindy Lou was treated by two physicians who told her that the small lump on her cervix was a viral wart disease. The physicians prescribed cream and told her she would be fine.

Cindy Lou began to have bleeding between periods and saw a third physician who happened to be experienced with DES-associated cancer. After requesting and reviewing the original slides and pathology reports, he found she had both venereal warts and cancer. The word *cancer* was something Cindy Lou couldn't bear to hear. She went to three different doctors hoping one of them would convince her that she did not have cancer. When all three confirmed the diagnosis, she returned to the physician who originally detected cancer and consented to surgery. Cindy Lou is only twenty-three years old. She will never be able to have a child, but she is alive today—and happy to be alive.

When the diagnosis is "cancer associated with DES," you will need surgery and possibly follow-up chemotherapy. Read the chapter on treatments (Chapter 11) and make a list of any questions you might have to discuss with your gynecologic oncology team. Remember, this is not a common cancer. Be certain you are with the best available team in your area. The surgery can be tricky and it is so extensive that it may require a plastic surgeon as well.

Under *no* circumstances should you consider preventive or prophylactic surgery—that is, surgery to treat the cancer before the cancer occurs. While it is difficult to document, some publications have talked about young women being treated with preventive surgery because their mothers took DES. Get a second opinion.

Get a third opinion. In fact, if preventive surgery is suggested to you at all, consider switching physicians immediately.

The surgery for DES-associated cancer is an abdominal radical hysterectomy. This involves removal of the cervix, the uterus, the upper part of the vagina, and the supporting structures. The ovaries are not automatically removed since they do not influence the cure and these patients are usually young. Be certain you discuss this with your physician beforehand so that he or she knows whether you want your ovaries left behind.

Sometimes when the upper part of the vagina is removed, a great deal of the vaginal structure must be taken out. Then an artificial vagina must be constructed. New plastic surgery techniques make this possible, but it may have to be done in a second, separate operation. (We discuss vaginal surgery in Chapter 9.) Because the plastic surgery techniques are new, you should have the initial operation done by a surgical team not only experienced in treating cases of vaginal cancer but also working in close cooperation with a proficient team of plastic surgeons. Women who undergo breast reconstruction often ask plastic surgeons for photographs of their work. You should ask a plastic surgeon what type of results you can expect from this type of surgery.

The prognosis for this type of cancer is quite good; surgery probably will cure you completely. Some women, however, will not receive treatment early enough. If you are not seen soon enough, you will need both surgery and chemotherapy to suppress the cells that have spread out of the pelvis. Because this is such a new disease, the results of chemotherapy are difficult to predict.

EMOTIONAL SIDE EFFECTS OF DES EXPOSURE

While there are frequently no problems with the surgery itself, the emotional trauma on young women who will never have the option to become mothers is often severe. For any type of surgery, it is important that you have some kind of emotional support. If your physician does not offer to have a liaison psychiatrist visit you after the surgery, ask for help from a cancer support group, and also check with DES Action. Professional help should be available and offered to you at the hospital, but if it is not, seek out a volunteer (particularly from DES Action) just to talk with you.

Women often feel depressed and need someone to talk to even after an uplifting experience such as giving birth. Assume that you will be relieved and happy and well after surgery, but don't play superwoman. Everyone needs a good listener after surgery of any kind—and surgery that leaves you sterile carries with it its own special problems.

The DES Task Force has suggested studies to determine the nature and extent of the psychosocial impact this problem has had, not just on women who took the drug but on their daughters as well. Those women who have been interviewed talk of feelings that range from guilt, to anger, to fear and a loss of self-image. DES mothers have noted particular difficulty with young daughters who are sexually inexperienced and frightened about the prospect of a pelvic exam.

The story that follows is significant for two reasons. The woman given DES received it in 1961, a full ten years after Congressional testimony regarding its dangers and after its effectiveness was questioned by the Chicago researchers. In addition, her daughter's experience, reminiscent of the dark ages of medicine, took place in the 1970s.

In 1976 Nadine Brozan of *The New York Times*, in reporting on DES mothers, told of a Long Island woman who reluctantly took DES in 1961. Today her worries are not just about her daughter's physical state, but about her emotional state as well.

"When my daughter had her first Pap smear at age eleven, she asked me, 'Mommy, is this what sex is like?'"

The mother went on to wonder what fears her daughter was

harboring and added, "The only way I have been able to get her to the doctor has been to cry and tell her, 'I would do this for you because I love you. Please do it for me because you love me.'"

If your daughter was exposed to DES *in utero* and is still young, there are several things you can do to minimize the trauma of her first pelvic exam. You might find her a woman physician with whom she might feel more comfortable. Or find a physician who uses anesthesia before examining a child. Or find a competent physician who is understanding, caring, and experienced. Since anesthesia always carries some risk, it is best to find a supportive and experienced gynecologist who can help ease the trauma of your child's first pelvic exam.

Take the time to interview the physician who will examine your child beforehand. Make certain that he or she is patient and understanding and has the type of personality that will have a calming, reassuring effect on your child. It is important—in fact, crucial—that a DES-exposed daughter be examined. It is not necessary, however, to subject her to a barbaric experience.

WHAT IS THE RISK FOR MOTHERS WHO TOOK DES?

Some studies indicate that DES mothers may be at an increased risk for breast cancer, but this has not yet been confirmed. Whether or not DES mothers are at an increased risk for gynecological cancer also has yet to be determined. The DES Task Force has recommended that DES mothers have an annual pelvic examination including a Pap smear and in addition undergo a breast examination that follows current National Cancer Institute guidelines for breast cancer screening. Those guidelines are:

- Monthly breast self-examination and the report of any abnormal findings to your physician.
- Annual palpation of the breasts by qualified medical personnel.

- No mammography under age thirty-five for routine screening.
- Between thirty-five and thirty-nine annual mammography only if you have a family history of breast cancer.

DES IN THE FOOD WE EAT

For many, many years, stilbesterol, also called DES, was used to fatten steers for market. Sometimes stilbesterol was put directly into the corn or other feed given to the animals; sometimes the chemical was placed under the skin of the animals. Stilbesterol increased the animals' weight, although this was due to an increase in fat and probably water retention rather than an increase in meat protein. It was not until 1979 that consumer groups succeeded in their efforts to keep DES (stilbesterol) out of the beef we eat. This ban, however, took thirty years to put into effect, for no one ever listened to the experts and learned from the mink lesson.

In the early 1950s, the use of DES nearly wiped out the then-sizable mink industry in America. To produce prized mink fur successfully, the animals needed high-grade protein foods. A government researcher suggested in the early 1950s that a palatable and cheap source of protein for minks would be discarded heads from commercially processed chickens.

Suddenly, disaster struck the mink farms. Two breeding seasons later, the fertility rate among minks had dropped almost to zero. Professor Robert K. Enders of Swarthmore College, a specialist in the biology of reproduction of animals, was called in to investigate the problem. Using biological sleuthing and having the cooperation of mink breeders who knew of his interest and talent, Dr. Enders found that the culprit was stilbesterol.

The chicken heads fed to the mink had come from "caponized" chickens. These chickens, *instead of having their male organs removed to make them plump and fat, had had a heavy dose of stilbesterol implanted in their necks.* The stilbesterol left in the chicken neck was absorbed by the minks and upset their finely tuned reproductive apparatus.

In 1951, in testimony before Congress, Dr. Enders warned of the hazards of DES. Although his students accepted his ideas, the government took no action on DES in human food. It took twenty years for DES to be banned in food.

Other studies pointed to the potential hazards of DES. Long before the attention of the public or the government was aroused to the potential problem, Professor William Gardner of Yale University proved that he could induce cancer with estrogenlike substances. As early as the 1930s, crude estrogen extracts were shown to be capable of inducing breast cancer in mice. By 1940, breast cancer was induced in rodents by putting stilbesterol in pellets under the skin. In the male mice in which the stilbesterol pellets were implanted, certain tumors of the testes were induced, possibly related to an upset in the natural hormonal control of that organ.

Tragically, despite these studies, no one said, "Stop, don't give this drug to women."

COULD A DES-TYPE TRAGEDY HAPPEN AGAIN?

Today we are a very test-conscious society. Through the efforts of consumer groups, consumer magazines, and Ralph Nader, we have become concerned for our safety. Suddenly women are demanding information; thirty years ago that was unheard of. They are more reluctant to turn over control of their bodies to physicians and prefer to work in partnership with them. But this attitude did not prevail in the 1940s and 1950s.

When women began asking their mothers, "Why didn't you question the doctor more carefully about DES?" what answers did they receive? "You did not question a doctor. You did as you were told!"

Despite what we have learned about DES, another medical tragedy could occur if women and physicians and researchers become lax about questioning the drugs that are on the market. With the use of anti-nausea drugs, it just may occur. Now we have the advantage of comparative studies that did not exist in the early 1940s, as well as the benefit of better-designed tests on drugs. But even now, we must not forget what happened with DES.

If you are a woman who cringes at the thought of questioning a doctor, remember some of the key aspects of the DES story: There were few comparative studies, despite the fact that the scientific literature of the time was filled with stories about the harmful effects of DES on animals. And despite the information the federal government had about the harm estrogen did to animals, we were permitted to consume DES in our beef and chicken for twenty years.

Whenever you are given a drug or medication or are treated with a new procedure, you should ask: How long has this drug been on the market? What type of tests have been done to determine its safety? How long were the tests continued? How many subjects were involved in the testing? Where are the stories from the opposition? What literature exists so that I can read about this myself? A good physician will be happy to direct you to the proper sources.

Librarians from local libraries will be able to help you with information about new drugs that have been publicized in the media. Your pharmacist will have information from his or her own journals which are usually not overly technical and can be a valuable source of information. Your physician, however, should be able to give you guidance, even if only to direct you to the hospital medical library to do your own research. If your physician is skeptical about your concern, remain undaunted. Make every effort to get every bit of information you need until you feel comfortable about the drug you are taking. If you sense that your physician is uncomfortable about your concern, find a physician with whom you can develop a working partnership in your own health care.

Chapter Five

The Uterus

When Gretchen was a young girl, she often said that she wanted to spend her life "barefoot and pregnant." She was in her early twenties when she married. Although she wanted to begin her family immediately, Gretchen had difficulty conceiving.

"I never knew what it was that caused my infertility. I do remember, however, that I had some kind of surgery. In those days we never asked the doctor many questions. He said 'Surgery'; I said 'Fine.' Actually the surgery was a success, because three months later I became pregnant," said Gretchen.

Eleven months after her first child was born, Gretchen again became pregnant. She wanted still a third child, but she began to have heavy and frequent periods that left her weak and fatigued. "With two little children and a near-constant period, I was exhausted. My large-family fantasy quickly faded," she said.

When her second baby was about three years old, Gretchen went for a routine gynecological exam. The physician told her that she had a hormone deficiency and a thyroid problem. "I took his word for it," she said. "He prescribed estrogen and a thyroid pill, which I took faithfully."

By the time Gretchen turned forty, she began to have periods heavier than she had ever before experienced. She decided to see a different specialist. The new physician spent time with her explaining what might be causing her heavy periods. He then suggested a D and C (dilation and curettage) with tissue analysis. The results showed that Gretchen had normal tissue of the uterine lining. Gretchen was told she had nothing to worry about; she was merely going through menopause.

For the next few years, Gretchen had no check-ups. During that time her periods stopped altogether. Then one day she noticed a slight bloody discharge. She had a bloody staining for about a week and decided to see her physician.

A biopsy of the endometrium—the mucous membrane that lines the uterus—was done in the physician's office. It revealed tissue that appeared to indicate endometrial cancer. Gretchen was hospitalized and had a D and C with further tissue analysis. Again the biopsy revealed abnormal tissue, the kind found in a precancerous condition called endometrial hyperplasia.

While there might be different treatments for hyperplasia, in Gretchen's case a hysterectomy was recommended. Today, four years later, she is considered completely cured.

When Eunice was twenty-eight years old and still childless, she and her husband decided to adopt a baby. Eunice had married at nineteen because she wanted to be the mother of ten children. "Can you imagine what it was like for me, when month after month went by and I didn't conceive?"

Eunice was actually relieved when she and her husband decided to adopt a baby but remembers those days as a time when she was "a bundle of nerves. I had always been on the heavy side, but during the adoption proceedings, I ate constantly. My blood pressure really shot up too," she recalled.

Eunice later learned, through tests at a fertility clinic, that she did not ovulate frequently. Her periods had always been irregular and infrequent. By the time she was thirty-six, they had stopped altogether. Five years later, when she was forty-two, she began to bleed heavily. The bleeding lasted for about two weeks. It was then that Eunice decided to go for her first check-up in three years. The physician hospitalized Eunice and did a D and C. Biopsy of the tissue revealed endometrial cancer. Eunice had a hysterectomy, which is curative treatment for very early cases. Today, six years later, she has had no recurrence of the disease.

Endometrial cancer, which usually strikes women between the ages of forty-five and sixty-five, affects about 38,000 women in the United States each year; that is, about one woman in every seventy. In the earliest stages, it is nearly 100 percent curable. For about 3,200 women, however, endometrial cancer will be fatal.

Although it is generally associated with menopause, some women develop endometrial cancer in their early thirties. If you have a condition called Stein-Leventhal syndrome, which is characterized by obesity, scanty periods or no periods at all, and infertility, you are also at greater risk.

WHAT IS THE ENDOMETRIUM?

The endometrium is the lining of the uterus. The uterus itself looks like an upside-down pear and usually is about the size of one. (Some women have a uterus as small as a plum, but this is not considered normal.) The cervix is the neck or narrow end of the uterus; the body of the organ is called the corpus.

The bleeding of menstruation is caused by the shedding of the endometrium. The lining of the uterus is under the control of ovarian hormones, which can be thought of as chemical messengers. These messenger hormones are sent by the ovaries to the uterus, which responds by growing in monthly cycles. At the end of the cycle, if you have not become pregnant, the lining will shed

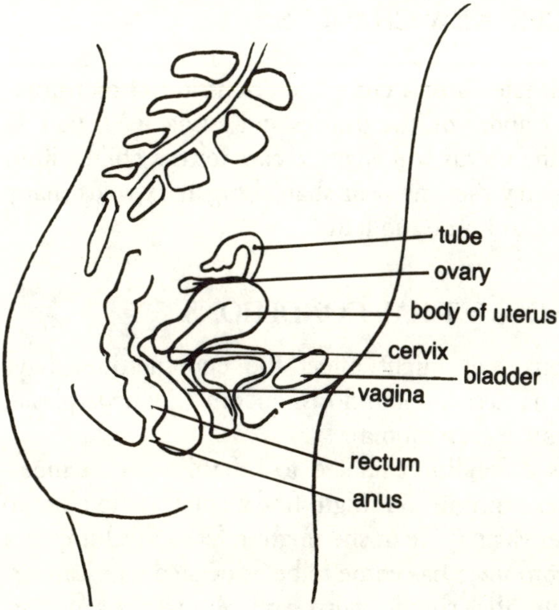

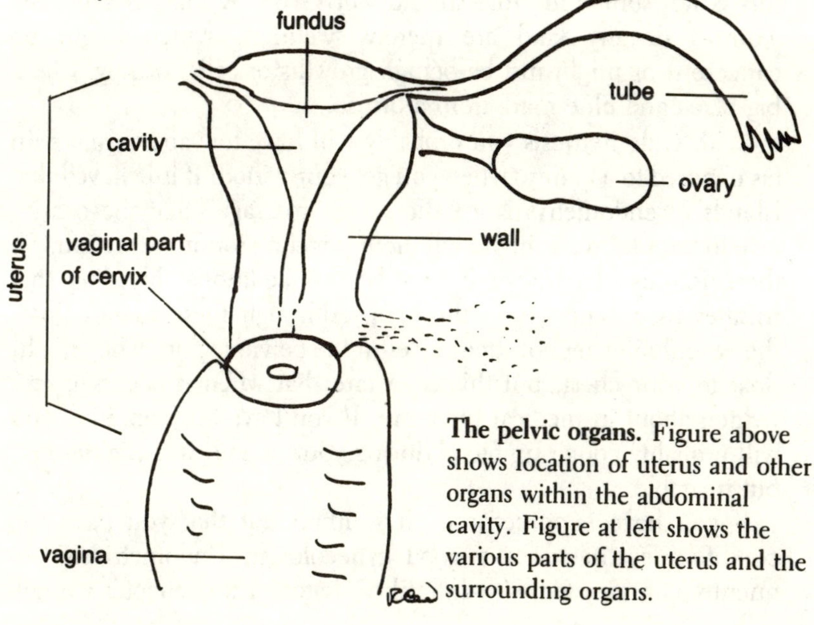

The pelvic organs. Figure above shows location of uterus and other organs within the abdominal cavity. Figure at left shows the various parts of the uterus and the surrounding organs.

and you will menstruate. (For a complete discussion of menstruation, see Chapters 7 and 8 on the ovaries and estrogen.) If you do become pregnant, the uterus will adapt to care for the child within you. During pregnancy the tiny pear-shaped organ expands many times its normal size to house the fetus.

ENDOMETRIAL CONDITIONS

Several conditions that might affect the endometrium have confusingly similar names: endometriosis, endometrial hyperplasia, and endometrial cancer (carcinoma).

Endometriosis is a condition related to infertility, not cancer. Your physician in examining you might find a small lump close to the cervix and upper vagina. He or she might refer to this lump as a mass. While the word *mass* has come to be associated with cancer, this is not something that should worry you. A mass is a tumor. Tumors of any kind are merely swellings, which might be cancerous or might just be benign growths of cells, or might be a big black and blue mark from a bruise.

With endometriosis you probably will have low abdominal pain (as opposed to a cramp) when you get your period. It is believed that islands of endometriosis get the same "message" that the ovaries give to the uterine lining to tell them it is time for menstruation. So these islands bleed also. It may be this additional bleeding that irritates tissue and causes the pain. Although these islands float, they eventually anchor themselves in the pelvic region. They might float to your chest, but this is so rare that when it occurs it gets written about in medical literature. If you have this condition you will probably cough up blood during your period. It is frightening, but treatable.

If you have endometriosis, it is important that you have the condition evaluated by a good gynecologist. Endometriosis frequently is associated with infertility. Later in this chapter we talk about infertility as a factor that puts women at a higher risk for endometrial cancer. Endometriosis has not been associated with cancer because in this case infertility is caused by a mechanical (tissue) blockage; infertility associated with cancer is a hormonal problem.

Endometrial hyperplasia and endometrial cancer are related conditions. Endometrial hyperplasia is called a precursor or forerunner to invasive endometrial cancer.

Hyperplasia literally means an overgrowth of tissue. If you have endometrial hyperplasia, also called adenomatous hyperplasia, too many cells have formed tissues in the lining of your uterus. How does this happen? The lining of the uterus is under the control of estrogen and progesterone, the hormones produced by the ovaries. It is at puberty that these hormones begin to interact during the menstrual and ovulation cycles.

Each month during your reproductive years, estrogen, which makes the lining of the uterus grow, is joined by another hormone, progesterone, produced by the ovaries after ovulation. Progesterone in combination with estrogen prepares the lining of the uterus for the implantation of a fertilized egg.

It is suspected that adenomateous hyperplasia is related to the failure of ovulation. If you do not ovulate, then only estrogen is produced in your body, and the balance of the two hormones is upset. The extra estrogen "unopposed" by progesterone stimulates or encourages the lining of the uterus to grow. When you keep producing estrogen, it thickens the uterine lining. In a woman who does not ovulate, the tissues of the lining of the uterus, when examined under a microscope, look somewhat like cancer. These tissues are not cancer, however; they constitute hyperplasia, an overgrowth of tissue that might continue to grow at a fast rate and might turn into a spreading cancer.

In addition to endometrial (adenomatous) hyperplasia, there is a special type called cystic glandular hyperplasia, which should be watched closely by your gynecologist. It is thought to be caused by lack of progesterone. It differs from adenomatous hyperplasia in that it does not appear to have the same predilection to become invasive cancer. It may, in fact, be the introductory phase to adenomatous hyperplasia but it requires little, if any, treatment.

Endometrial hyperplasia appears to affect women who have a high-risk cancer profile or "triad": They are extremely overweight, have diabetes, and have high blood pressure. Just how overweight is overweight? The American Cancer Society has said that women who are 40 percent overweight have a mortality rate five-and-one-half times as high as that of average-weight women. This means that if you should weigh 100 pounds, but weigh 140 pounds instead, you are seriously overweight and are putting yourself at an increased risk for endometrial cancer. Put another way, a 1980 American Cancer Society Report noted that in 1966, Dr. Ernst Wynder of the American Health Foundation found that women twenty-one to fifty pounds overweight were about three times as likely as women who were of normal or below-normal weight to develop endometrial cancer, and those women who were fifty pounds overweight were ten times as likely to develop endometrial cancer.

In addition to the conditions of overweight, hypertension (high blood pressure), and diabetes, you might be considered at high risk for endometrial cancer if you are still single in midlife, have never been pregnant, are infertile, have had irregular periods most of your life, and have been taking certain estrogen pills.

A Denver pathologist has suggested that certain endometrial cancers in younger women are related to the use of oral contraceptives *(The New England Journal of Medicine*, vol. 302, 1980) but may act differently. Because of this, some physicians are questioning whether or not it is the same type of endometrial cancer as is found in older women.

The most hotly debated issue has been the use of estrogen to relieve the symptoms of menopause. Studies have shown that women taking what are called exogenous hormones, such as Premarin, are at an increased risk for endometrial cancer. One study was originally reported in *The New England Journal of Medicine* and then refuted several months later. (A complete discussion of the pros and cons of estrogen therapy is in Chapter 8.) You should be aware, however, that the National Cancer Institute noted in a special communication of May 22, 1978, "For some women the cancer risk associated with estrogen may outweigh its benefit as a means of relieving symptoms of menopause. Studies have shown that women taking estrogen for menopausal symptoms have roughly 5 to 10 times greater chance of developing uterine cancer as women who take no estrogen."

Symptoms

Bleeding is the most common symptom of endometrial hyperplasia and cancer. Although women who develop this type of cancer often have infrequent periods, an unusually heavy period is worth investigating. There are office procedures that physicians can perform to detect endometrial hyperplasia or cancer, but the best means of detection for women is their own self-awareness. If you are aware of your periods and your monthly menstrual cycle, you might well spot the symptoms of cancer or its precursor at its earliest and most treatable stage. Excessive bleeding is almost always an indicator that something is amiss within your body.

How well do you know your body and its monthly cycle?

- How long is your menstrual cycle? Twenty-four days? Twenty-eight days? Thirty-three days?
- What kind of menstrual flow do you have? Light? Heavy?
- How long a period do you generally have? Three days? Eight days or longer?
- Are you very uncomfortable during your periods? That is, do you have cramping backaches?

If you know about your periods and how you experience them, when a change occurs you can intelligently discuss it with your physician. What type of changes should you be aware of?

• Increase in the frequency of your periods; that is, instead of having a twenty-eight-day cycle, which is normal for you, you begin to bleed every twenty days instead.

• Increase in quantity of the flow itself. If you usually have heavy bleeding on the first day, then that may be normal for you. If, however, you find that you are flowing so heavily that you are spending two or three days in bed, see a physician.

• Increase in the number of days that you normally flow; that is, if you suddenly go from bleeding five days to bleeding eight or ten, that might be an indication of a serious problem.

• Increase in significant pain during menstruation.

Any of these changes in your periods may indicate endometrial hyperplasia or endometrial cancer. Clotting and/or bleeding may be perfectly normal during menopause, but each can also be a symptom of cancer. Do not dismiss heavy bleeding as a menopause problem.

Testing Conditions

A physician may use several different types of procedures to check you for endometrial hyperplasia or cancer. In each case, confirmation is made through tissue analysis of the cells removed from the endometrium. The cells can be extracted through an endometrial aspiration biopsy or similar technique. This test can be done during a routine office visit. Another method for determining the presence of abnormal cells is a D and C; this procedure is most often performed in a hospital but can be done in a physician's office as well.

If you are given an endometrial aspiration biopsy, the entire procedure will take only a few minutes. First, the walls of the vagina are opened with a speculum. Then a metal tube about half the thickness of a drinking straw is inserted into the cervix. Tissue is sucked out and sent to a pathologist for review. Within two or three days you will have a diagnosis.

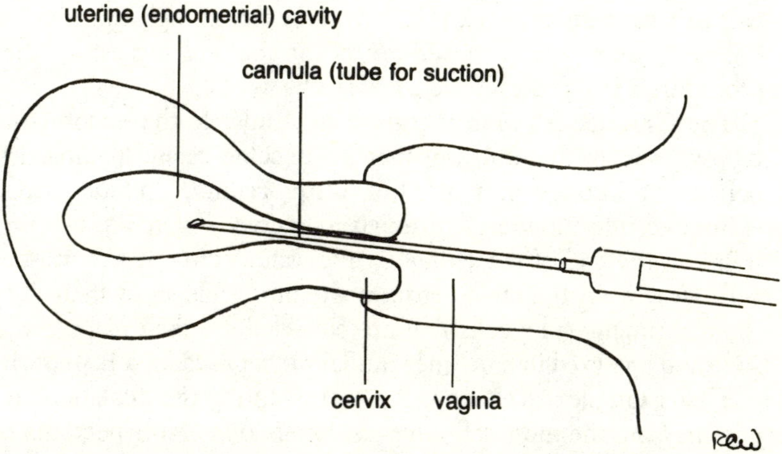

Endometrial aspiration biopsy. A metal tube is inserted into the cervix. When the physician squeezes a rubber bulb at the end of the tube, tissue from the uterine lining is sucked up. This material is then sent to a pathologist for review.

The major drawback to the aspiration procedure is pain and possibly some cramping. There are many nerve endings in the cervix, and because the cervix itself is rigid, insertion of a metal tube hurts.

Since the aspiration biopsy can indicate so dependably the presence of abnormal cells, many gynecologic oncologists think it should be done routinely on every office visit. Most physicians, however, shy away from doing the test routinely, reasoning that women who are already edgy about a pelvic exam might be discouraged altogether from regular check-ups if a painful procedure is involved. The test will add $10 to $20 to your office exam cost.

The decision to have an endometrial biopsy is really yours. If you are a high-risk person, then you should consider making the test a part of your regular check-ups. If you are not at high risk, discuss this with your physician; perhaps he or she will suggest another procedure such as the Gravelee jet wash.

The Gravelee jet wash is somewhat similar to the endometrial biopsy. It is less painful, but many gynecologists and pathologists believe it is also less accurate. For this procedure, a plastic syringe is inserted into the uterus, through the cervix. There are two tiny holes on the end of the syringe; while water from one side washes cells away from the endometrium, the other side sucks them into the instrument. The cells that are collected are then placed on a slide and analyzed in a manner similar to that used for a Pap smear.

Tissue samples taken from the uterus during the dilatation and curettage are the most definitive test for endometrial hyperplasia or cancer. If office biopsies indicate the presence of abnormal or cancerous cells, a good gynecologist will perform a D and C before prescribing treatment.

Conventional D and Cs are done in a hospital using general or local anesthesia. Usually an overnight stay is required, but some women stay just for the day. There is frequently no pain involved in a D and C and you can expect to be fully active soon after the procedure.

There are also D and Cs that can be performed in a physician's office for diagnosing endometrial problems. Procedures for an office D and C differ slightly from hospital procedures. In an office, a physician is most likely to use a suction type of device, such as a Vabra, which is another hollow metal tube with suction supplied by a pump. Office D and Cs are performed using local anesthesia, and there is some discomfort.

Should you have a D and C performed in a hospital or in a

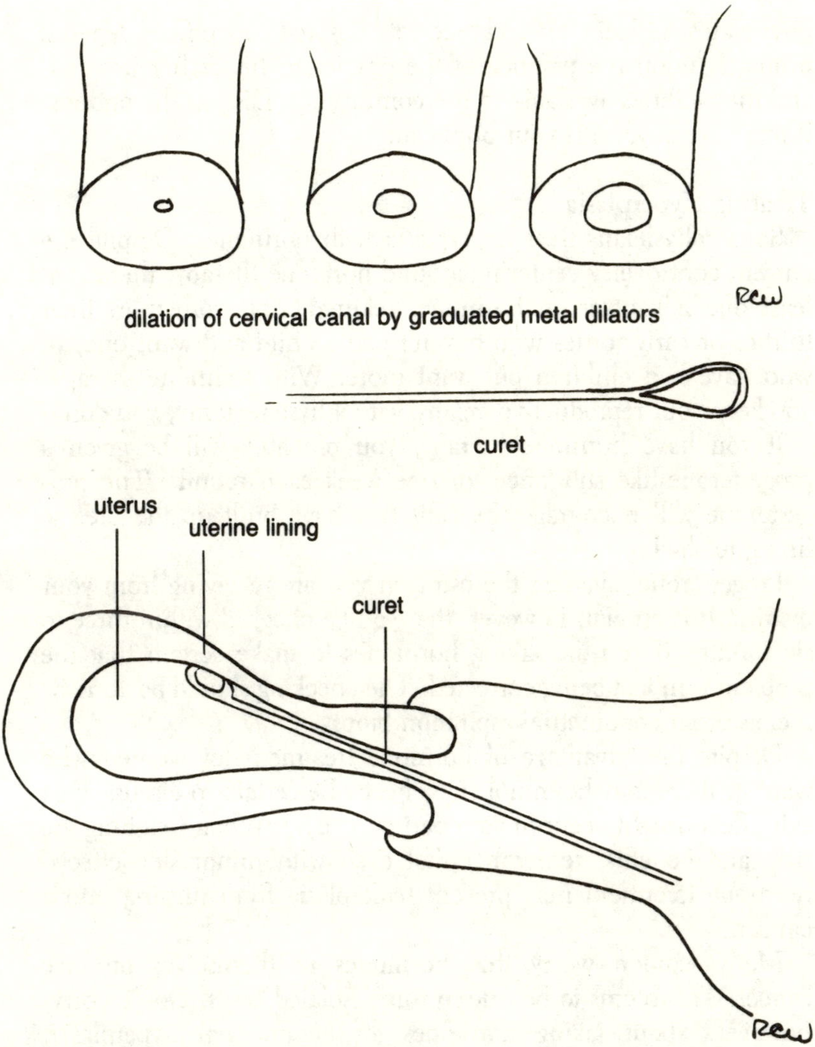

Dilatation and curettage. The cervical canal is dilated by use of graduated metal rods, called dilators. The spoon-shaped metal curet is used to scrape away a portion of the uterine lining.

physician's office? The choice of hospital or office depends primarily upon the practice of the physician, his or her hospital, and the facilities available in the community. Discuss the options, if there are any, with your physician.

Treating Hyperplasia

Some physicians treat hyperplasia with hormones. Despite the current controversy centering around hormone therapy, there is at least one advantage to hormone treatment for women in their thirties or early forties who haven't had a child and want one, or who have had children but want more. With hormone therapy, you keep your reproductive organs; with a hysterectomy, you don't.

If you have hormone therapy, you probably will be given a progesterone-like substance for one week each month. The progesterone will encourage the cells that have built up the uterine lining to shed.

Progesterone balances the estrogen you are receiving from your ovaries. It is crucial, however, that you be checked within three to six months if you are taking hormones to make certain that the problem is in fact being corrected. The checking should be done by means of an endometrial aspiration biopsy.

Despite the advantage of hormone treatment for women who want it, there may be minor side effects. Be certain to discuss what side effects might occur in your particular case. When weighing the risks and benefits, remember that even with minor side effects, hormone treatment may prevent hyperplasia from turning into a cancer.

Many women worry that hormones in themselves produce cancer. This seems to be true in some isolated cases. Don't worry, however, about taking hormones for endometrial hyperplasia. Why? Because the hormone used is like progesterone. This has *never* been associated with those that induce cancer.

If you fit the high-risk profile for endometrial cancer, if your mother had endometrial cancer or if you have hyperplasia, and if you don't want any more children, your physician will most likely suggest a hysterectomy as treatment. This is because your chances of developing cancer increase if you have hyperplasia.

If a hysterectomy is suggested, you will be admitted to the hospital, probably a day or two before the surgery. (See Chapter 11 for a complete discussion of preoperative tests and postoperative convalescence.) For hyperplasia, you will have what is called a total or complete hysterectomy, which is removal of the cervix and the corpus, the body of the uterus. Removal of the ovaries and tubes is not necessary for treatment of hyperplasia.

ENDOMETRIAL CANCER

Endometrial cancer may run in families. No one is certain whether there is a genetic predisposition to endometrial cancer. It may simply be that women whose mothers had endometrial cancer are more aware of it and therefore more likely to seek help when they spot symptoms in their own cases.

Mildred's mother had serious "female problems." "In those days," said Mildred, "anything at all relating to periods or menopause was called 'female trouble.' My mother fit the high-risk cancer profile for endometrial cancer, and even though I knew she died of cancer, I never realized it was endometrial cancer until I questioned her doctor some years later. He alerted me to the symptoms."

Four years after her own menopause, Mildred began to bleed heavily. Recalling her mother's experience, she went immediately to a gynecologist. "I had him put me right into the hospital for a D and C. I wasn't taking any chances," she said.

Mildred was hospitalized, and analysis of the tissue from the D and C did reveal invasive cancer. She had a hysterectomy, as well as radiation treatments and is alive today, six years after treatment. Although Mildred went to a physician immediately, her cancer had already begun to spread. It was for this reason that she underwent surgery and follow-up radiation.

Anna spent years taking care of her widowed mother Concetta. She never married, never became pregnant, and had infrequent periods most of her life. Less than eight years after her mother had surgery for endometrial cancer, Anna was found to have the disease as well. She was treated, and today, ten years later, she is considered cured.

There is an irony, however, in Anna's mother's case. Concetta was sixty pounds overweight, had high blood pressure, and was diabetic. Although she fit the high-risk profile, she did not have any ovaries; they had been removed shortly after the birth of her daughter. What, then, was it that could have caused endometrial cancer? Some researchers have suggested that in severely overweight women, a process called peripheral conversion takes place in fatty tissue whereby substances such as cholesterol are turned into estrogen. Cholesterol in the body is called a precursor to estrogen because a cholesterol molecule can be changed (through certain metabolic processes) into an estrogen precursor and then into estrogen itself. In Concetta's case, excess estrogen seemed to be the result of her overweight.

Endometrial cancer, like hyperplasia, is believed to be the result of an overproduction of estrogen. When ovulation does not occur, no progesterone is produced to balance the estrogen made by the ovaries. This situation appears to create a climate for endometrial cancer.

In general, if you have had irregular menstrual cycles throughout your life, you have a greater chance of having hyperplasia. If you have hyperplasia that remains untreated, your chances of developing cancer increase.

Hyperplasia will develop into cancer in about 15 to 20 percent of all cases. While it is usually possible to detect the changes, there are rare cases in which the change from hyperplasia to cancer takes place so rapidly that it seems as if the cancer started without an intervening step. But there is no way to be certain whether or not this is the case. There are even some rare cases where a precursor does not develop and the cancer springs into existence without a latent phase.

With endometrial cancer, you will probably have symptoms such as an extremely heavy period or bleeding between periods. A biopsy from tissues obtained during a D and C is the most important test for definitive confirmation of endometrial cancer. When there is a strong possibility that you have endometrial cancer, because of symptoms and/or because you are a high-risk person, and test results from an office biopsy show cancerous cells, you will probably go into the hospital for the D and C. Some physicians will suggest you remain in the hospital while the tissue is analyzed. If the test results show cancer, you will most likely receive preoperative radiation treatment two or three days later. Surgery often follows in a few days, say, about six days after first entering the hospital. If you want a second opinion, it would be best to get it immediately after analysis of the tissue obtained from the D and C. In this case you might simply request that your physician seek the opinion of two different pathologists.

In preoperative radiation, the first step in treating endometrial cancer, tiny capsules are placed in the uterus. They are about the size of vitamin pills and are filled with radium, cobalt, cesium, or some similar radioactive substance. The purpose is to shrink the tumor and devitalize the cancer cells.

You may be in a hospital center that uses external radiation (for a complete discussion of external radiation and its side effects, see Chapter 11). Depending on the size of the tumor and its location in the uterus, both internal and external radiation may be used. This is *not* a frequent occurrence. The side effects of external radiation are slightly more severe than those of internal radiation treatment.

After a few days, your physician usually will decide that the tumor has shrunk enough for a hysterectomy to be performed—a total abdominal hysterectomy and bilateral salpingo-oophorectomy. A total abdominal hysterectomy, TAH, is removal of the uterus; bilateral salpingo-oophorectomy (BSO) means removal of the fallopian tubes, called salpingectomy, and removal of the ovaries, called oophorectomy. Once cancer invades an organ (as opposed to being confined to specific layers of tissue), the chances that some cells have spread to surrounding organs increases. Also, if the ovaries were to remain and keep on producing estrogen, they might stimulate residual cancer cells that have traveled elsewhere in the body.

It is possible that your physician will consider a vaginal hysterectomy. This is not commonly used for treatment of cancer. Although you might prefer this type of surgery, which leaves less of a scar, it is not advisable. From a technical point of view, it is difficult for the surgeon to remove the ovaries and tubes through a vaginal incision, and, with endometrial cancer, you do not want your ovaries left behind.

Once the ovaries have been removed, you will experience what some women think is the most uncomfortable side effect of treatment for endometrial cancer—surgical menopause. With surgical menopause you are likely to experience symptoms of estrogen withdrawal, such as hot flashes, vaginal dryness, and irritability. Because endometrial cancer is an estrogen-sensitive tumor, estrogen cannot be given to alleviate these symptoms: Any hidden cancer might be stimulated by the hormone.

Many women do not experience estrogen withdrawal symptoms. If you do need a drug to alleviate symptoms, however, there are substitutes, marketed drugs, none of which give as much relief as estrogen. (Whether or not you should ever take estrogen to relieve menopausal symptoms is being seriously questioned today; see Chapter 8.)

Another treatment is used today for endometrial cancer; it is called hormonal therapy. If hormonal therapy is suggested, it is because cancer has already spread beyond the body of the uterus. Although this is not a symptomless disease and advanced detection methods are available, there are rare instances in which there are no symptoms and an advanced tumor is discovered during a routine office visit. Sometimes it is treatable with surgery, but sometimes surgery would not be curative and hormonal therapy is used. In addition to hormonal therapy, today there are new treatments, especially chemotherapeutic agents, that appear to offer long-term control of the disease.

RELATED ENDOMETRIAL CONDITIONS: POLYPS AND FIBROIDS

Endometrial polyps are tiny fingerlike projections that grow on the endometrium. They may produce the same symptoms as endometrial hyperplasia or cancer, that is, bleeding between periods or extremely heavy bleeding at the time of your period. While you should see a physician to determine what is causing the bleeding, a diagnosis of polyps should not worry you a great deal. Polyps are easily removed through either a scraping or a D and C. After removal of the polyps, you should discuss with your physician your cancer risk and whether or not you should follow up with endometrial aspiration biopsies on a regular basis.

Fibroids (benign growths) affect 50 percent of all women.

Fibroids often regress slightly at the menopause but those that grow too large, perhaps to the size of a grapefruit or melon, are removed surgically. (See Chapter 7 on ovaries.)

If you have fibroids, the use of a sonar machine will help your physician to "watch" them. Fibroids do not predispose you to cancer. There is, however, a malignant variety of fibroid called leiomyosarcomas. This kind of fibroid is usually found only in older women, and it is extremely rare, occurring in just one of every 800 or 1,000 cases.

Do not let fear of this rare type of fibroid cancer scare you into surgery. If you have a fibroid that is being watched carefully by your physician, then you should not be overly concerned about it. It is only when an already existing fibroid begins to grow very suddenly and very rapidly that you should have immediate treatment. The usual treatment is surgery.

PREVENTING ENDOMETRIAL CANCER

Because researchers are beginning to understand better the relationship between diet and cancer, it may be that a special diet can be devised for women who are at high risk of developing endometrial cancer. The area of nutrition offers hope. The National Cancer Institute, while acknowledging an apparent relationship between obesity and cancer of the endometrium and of the breast, has noted that full-scale studies of that relationship have not yet been performed.

If obesity provides the excess fatty tissue where conversion of cholesterol to cancer-forming estrogen takes place, then control of obesity, however difficult, would be a means to prevent this cancer. While it would be irresponsible to say, "Today we *know* that you can prevent endometrial cancer through proper diet," we *can* say that you should consider a serious weight-loss program if you are a high-risk person. Serious overweight, high blood pressure, and even diabetes can be managed through proper nutrition.

It is also believed that the high blood pressure in the endometrial cancer triad is caused by excess overweight. Even if high blood pressure itself is only a contributing cause of endometrial cancer, then reducing that pressure would be a means of controlling the cancer risk. Through certain salt-restrictive diets and exercise, high blood pressure can be controlled.

If it is determined that endometrial cancer is a genetic problem, then until such time as genetic engineering is perfected, there will be no way to prevent the disease. But even women with genetic predisposition to cancer can be carefully watched and should be aware of symptoms.

Awareness of symptoms of endometrial hyperplasia and cancer is a choice available to all women. Learn about your menstrual cycles so the minute you detect a symptom that might indicate cancer, you can get help. Remember: In the precursor stage, your chance for complete cure after treatment is close to 100 percent.

RARE UTERINE CANCERS

Choriocarcinoma

Perhaps the strangest of all malignancies that affect the uterus—as well as one of the rarest—is choriocarcinoma, cancer of the placenta. It is far more common in Mexico, the Philippines, Taiwan and other parts of Asia than it is in North America, and it has been associated with poor protein intake and malnutrition. Chorio (pronounced CORE-e-o) is generally found in younger women of child-bearing age. Its early symptoms mimic pregnancy; in fact, the diagnosis is usually made on the basis of abnormally high levels of HCG (human gonadotropin), the pregnancy hormone, which is made by both a normal placenta and by this malignant tumor.

Choriocarcinoma is one of a group of disorders called trophoblastic disease. This group also includes hydatid or hydatiform mole. When this condition—also extremely rare—occurs, the uterus becomes filled with a large cluster of grape-like vesicles (hydatid means drop-like or grape-like) which replace the placenta and no baby develops. Hydatid mole (in many cases) makes the uterus grow larger than a normal pregnancy would, and when no heartbeat can be heard, the physician should suspect this disease. A diagnosis can be made easily with sonar and by measuring the levels of HCG in the blood and urine.

When choriocarcinoma is suspected or known, you should find a specialist with experience in treating this disease.

The first part of the treatment is usually a D & C (dilation and curettage). If the tumor in the uterus is the only one in the body, the HCG level should drop and return to normal in about a month's time. You should continue to be checked regularly and, if no HCG levels are found after one year, you may again try to become pregnant.

Sometimes the level of HCG remains high or rises even after the D & C. In this case, chemotherapy with actinomycin-D or methotrexate will be necessary. These two drugs have proved astonishingly successful in curing the disease in its early stages. With chemotherapy, the uterus can be saved—and along with it a woman's child-bearing capacity. It is very important, though, that these drugs be carefully monitored by someone experienced in their use. Both can have very serious side effects.

If the disease has existed for more than a few months, if ineffective treatment has been given, or if the disease has already spread to the liver or brain, the outlook is less promising. Patients are treated with methotrexate, actinomycin-D, and a third drug, usually cytoxan. Even in this more advanced stage, though, the chance of cure remains relatively good. In fact, choriocarcinoma was the first disease to be cured by chemotherapy in the twentieth century.

There are some choriocarcinomas—rarer still— that arise without pregnancy. They arise in the ovary (they can also occur in men, in the testes) and can be treated with the same three drugs, though the outcome might not be as good. For the majority of women with trophoblastic disease, though, a complete cure may be anticipated.

Sarcoma

Malignant tumors arising from the lining of organs and from their surfaces are usually in the group called carcinomas, or more commonly, cancers. But there are other, rare tumors that arise from within the walls of organs and from parts of the body that have no lining. These are called sarcomas. In the female genital tract, sarcomas may arise from fatty tissue under the skin of the vulva; in the wall of the uterus, in the ovary, or in the supporting tissues of any part of the genital tract. The sarcomas of greatest clinical significance are those that arise in the uterus and the vagina.

Most sarcomas of the genital tract arise in the uterus itself, usually in middle-aged or older women. (They can occur in women of any age, though, and even in little girls.) Abnormal bleeding sometimes brings the tumor to attention. Occasionally, a simple gynecological examination will reveal an enlargement that is later found to be a sarcoma. Unfortunately, some of these tumors escape detection until they have spread widely.

A combination of surgery and radiation used to be the standard approach for sarcomas. Nowadays, though, chemotherapy is more and more likely to be used after the tumor is surgically removed. If detected early enough, before the disease has spread, sarcomas can be cured, or at least controlled for a long period of time. The story of Mary Ellen is a lesson in how *not* to approach this disease.

Mary Ellen had come to the United States from her Carribbean home after the second World War. She settled in Pittsburgh and did domestic work until, at 60, her arthritis and obesity forced her to retire. She lived with cousins who looked after her. She could not remember exactly when her menopause had occurred, but she knew it had been ten to fifteen years earlier, so she was distressed to have an episode of bleeding. Her physician suggested an immediate curettage, but Mary Ellen refused—until a second episode brought her to the emergency room. She underwent curettage and was diagnosed as having a uterine sarcoma.

Mary Ellen underwent a hysterectomy; her tubes and ovaries were removed as well. Doctors wanted to do follow-up chemotherapy, but Mary Ellen was unwilling to make the repeated trips to either a hospital or a doctor's office for treatments and blood counts. Finally, a team of doctors convinced her to go to a hospital close to her home. She started treatments, but her attendance record for her treatments and the blood counts has been poor. Mary Ellen has taken the attitude that chemotherapy isn't worth the trouble.

And that's too bad, because chemotherapy has eliminated the hopelessness once felt for sarcoma. Cure rates for sarcoma are not quite so good as for choriocarcinoma—which is curable in most cases—but effective treatment is available. It's not likely that you will develop either of these two rare types of cancer, but if you do, the outlook is good.

Chapter Six

The Breast

Did you ever notice what happens to a woman when she begins discussing breast cancer with someone? Her hands instinctively reach upward and she brushes each breast with her hands. "Yes, they are both there," you can almost hear her saying to herself.

Phoebe was only thirty-four when she accidentally discovered that she had breast cancer. "I woke up one bright and glorious morning, thrilled to be in this wonderful new apartment of mine," she said. "I reached out as if to catch the sunbeams that woke me, stretched, hugged myself as I danced around the room, and felt something hard and curious in my breast. My arm hit it first. I stopped and, like a magnet, my hand went right to this tiny, hard spot. Instinctively, I knew it was cancer. I can still remember how calmly I called my brother-in-law, a surgeon, to tell him. I was afraid, not so much of losing my breast, but my life. I guess I was fortunate; my cancer was discovered at a very early stage, back in—let me see—I guess it was the summer of 1944, nearly 40 years ago.

"You know," added Phoebe, "in many ways it was much easier for us emotionally than it is for women today. There were no alternative treatments, no choice between radiation or surgery. I knew a number of women in my day who had their breasts removed, only then we didn't discuss it. In some ways, maybe it was easier."

Carla was just thirty-eight when she discovered a small lump in her breast. Although she was an intelligent, well-educated woman, she did not seek immediate treatment. Carla's breast cancer occurred at a time when newer detection and treatment methods were often discussed in the media. "When it happens to you," she said, "you're in such shock, it is almost too difficult to face it."

Carla waited three months before seeking treatment. By that time, she had to undergo breast removal and also receive follow-up chemotherapy.

In the early 1980s, the incidence of breast cancer was reported to be increasing. In 1979, it was estimated that approximately one in every thirteen baby girls born would eventually develop breast cancer; by 1980 that figure is being put at one in every eleven. The expected number of newly diagnosed cases in women will be approximately 100,000 this year. For about 37,000 women, the disease will be fatal. With a disease that has so many different detection methods, these fatality figures are too high.

The sooner cancer is detected, the more likely it is that it can be cured. New detection methods make it possible to find lumps so small that they cannot even be felt. In such cases, treatment may be very simple. The American Cancer Society reports an 85 percent cure rate. Some physicians report survival rates (meaning patients who live five years or more) of as much as 90 percent if the treatments are begun early enough. The trouble is that only one-half of breast cancers are detected when they are at this early, easily treatable stage.

Because of late detection, most women who are found to have the disease will undergo removal of the breast. The drastic step of breast removal—mastectomy—has to be taken in so many cases in order to prevent cancer from spreading. If left alone, cancer will continue to invade, that is, spread to the lymph nodes and other parts of the body.

Fatalities from breast cancer could be lower if more women regularly examined themselves or had their physicians examine them. In 1980, a survey by the American Cancer Society showed that only 24 percent of the women interviewed were examining their own breasts on a monthly basis. Another 1980 survey—by the National Institutes of Health—came up with a higher figure: 40 percent. But even the high figure is far lower than the ideal, considering that such examinations are easily done, take only a few minutes of your time, and may save your life.

THE BREAST

Breasts give femininity; they make women feel like women. Technically, breasts are highly specialized secretory organs. In a woman, they consist of milk-producing glands as well as fat.

When a teenager makes the transition from childhood to womanhood, estrogen production causes her breasts to change in shape. They become larger and fuller. The process usually begins when a young girl is between the ages of nine and thirteen.

Although breasts vary in size and shape, all are essentially mounds of gland-containing fat covered by skin. The nipple is in the middle of a darkened area called the *areola*. Sometimes nipples rise slightly above the areola, and sometimes they don't. The areola may be smooth, but usually it has tiny bumps called Montgomery's tubercles. The milk-producing glands within the breast increase in size during pregnancy.

Some women believe that during menstruation their breasts get bigger; this is because their breasts feel tender and puffy due to fluid retention. Changes take place within the breast during the menstrual cycle as the breasts react to the hormones produced. During various times in the cycle, lumps may be present that disappear afterward.

Some women always have lumps, these are women with benign cystic mastitis—a noncancerous condition also called fibrocystic disease. Lumps in the breast are very common, although some of them may be early cancer.

NONCANCEROUS BREAST CONDITIONS

Lumps in the breast might be the result of common breast diseases; one such is cystic mastitis (fibrocystic disease). With some types of cystic breast disease, there may be a greater risk for developing cancer.

With cystic mastitis, there are usually multiple lumps. Women with cystic mastitis report that symptoms include a full, tender feeling. Sometimes there will be a dull, heavy pain. These symptoms are more pronounced just before menstruation.

Most women who have large, uncomfortable breast lumps have them removed surgically. Even after surgery, new lumps often appear. A simpler approach to breast lump reduction has been suggested.

As early as 1965, Dr. Archie A. Abrams of the Boston University School of Medicine reported relief for premenstrual women and the reduction in cysts from the use of vitamin E. Later, in 1979, it was determined in a study funded by the American Cancer Society that many—but not all—women who received 600 units of vitamin E had noticeable improvement, and in some cases the lumps disappeared completely. This was reported in the *Journal of the American Medical Association*.

Some women with cystic mastitis can also reduce or eliminate breast lumps by following the regime of Dr. John Peter Minton, of the Department of Surgery at Ohio State University College of

Medicine. Dr. Minton's prescription: Do away with coffee, tea, cola, and chocolate—substances that contain xanthine derivative. These substances may stimulate formation of fibrous tissue and cyst fluid through cell growth. He also advises women to stop smoking.

These lumps usually come about through the build-up of breast tissue. Removal of the lump is usually necessary to exclude the possibility of cancer. Sometimes the ducts become plugged and the result is a cystic swelling. To determine whether or not these lumps are malignant, a physician might draw fluid or tissue with a thin needle from the cyst or lump and have it analyzed. This is called a needle aspiration biopsy.

Fibromas, sometimes called fibroadenomas, are another type of breast lump. They are also referred to as fibroids. They are found most often in younger women, although anyone from ages fifteen to forty can have one. Fibroadenomas are firm, nontender nodules, which grow in breast tissue and sometimes are confused with a true cancer on a simple physical examination. Mammography is the most often used method in distinguishing between fibromas and cancer.

Treatment for fibromas is usually surgery, but surgery is not always necessary. Although fibromas do not become cancerous tissue, some women have them removed to reassure themselves that they do not have cancer. Another reason that fibromas are removed is because they sometimes get very large. Occasionally, when a mammogram confirms a small fibroma, and the physician watches to see that it is not growing, watching and waiting are sufficient.

WHO IS AT RISK FOR BREAST CANCER?

In addition to those with benign breast lumps, all women over the age of twenty-five are at risk for breast cancer. Among those aged forty to forty-four, it is the leading cause of death.

The incidence of breast cancer above the age of forty is higher in women who never marry. For example, some studies show an excessive mortality rate from breast cancer among Catholic nuns.

Women who marry and have their first full-term pregnancy before the age of twenty have less risk of breast cancer than women who are first pregnant at age thirty-five or older. Also at less risk are women who have had four or more children as compared with just one child. The association with high parity, while shown in some studies, is nevertheless not as consistent as the effect of an early age at the first live birth.

Breast cancer does tend to "run" in families, and the risk is especially high if the cancer was diagnosed premenopausally or bilaterally. Your risk for developing breast cancer is two to three times greater if you have close relatives with breast cancer. If your mother or sisters have had breast cancer, your risk may be still higher. If cancer has appeared in your family, you must make this clear to your physicians. Once considered far-fetched, the theory that breast cancer and even some other cancers run in families has been studied and documented for a number of years. There *is* a genetically related risk.

If you had breast cancer in one breast, your chance of developing breast cancer in the second breast is *five times* greater than if you never had breast cancer. Also at greater risk for breast cancer are women who have had treatment for ovarian and endometrial cancer (cancer of the lining of the uterus).

Nor can the link between diet and cancer be ignored. If you are overweight and have a high fat intake, you might be at high risk for the disease. The link between diet and cancer is explored at the end of this chapter in the section on cause and prevention.

High-risk women—all women, in fact—should not only be aware of detection methods, but also use them. When it comes to breast cancer detection, the first responsibility is yours!

DETECTION AND TREATMENT

The single most important method of detecting breast disease, including cancer, is BSE—breast self-examination. Many women consider BSE "looking for trouble." Yet for those women who have indeed found lumps and received prompt medical attention, breast self-examination has been a lifesaver. Why is it that in the United States, where there is one death from breast cancer almost every fifteen minutes, 60 percent of the women do not practice the simple procedure that can help keep them from becoming a statistic? The following stories are typical:

Janine is the acquisitions editor of a large women's magazine. She has been in the business "for as long as I can remember." When the interest in women's issues surfaced, she was on the West Coast. Recognizing a trend about to blossom, Janine became particularly interested in articles submitted to her concerning women's health. "Whenever I saw a story on breast examinations, however, I shuddered," she said. "I have always had a tendency to cystic mastitis. I tried examining my breasts for a while, but everytime I found a lump, it made me nervous. After a while, I just stopped bothering to check."

Carrie is convinced that breast self-examinations are the best thing that ever happened for women. "But I just haven't managed to get into a routine. Besides, I'm not really at the high-risk stage yet. When I hit thirty-five, I'll get more organized."

Kathy is fifty-three. She is the mother of four children and owns her own specialty shop and her own bookshop. "Breast self-examination? I've been fine all these years; I'm not going to start looking for trouble now!"

The guidelines recommended by the American Cancer Society suggest a breast self-examination for every woman over the age of twenty. It is simple, easy, and 100 percent safe. The following pictures and text are from the American Cancer Society booklet (2203 LE).

HOW TO EXAMINE YOUR BREASTS

1 In the shower: Examine your breasts during bath or shower; hands glide easier over wet skin. Fingers flat, move gently over every part of each breast. Use right hand to examine left breast, left hand for right breast. Check for any lump, hard knot or thickening.

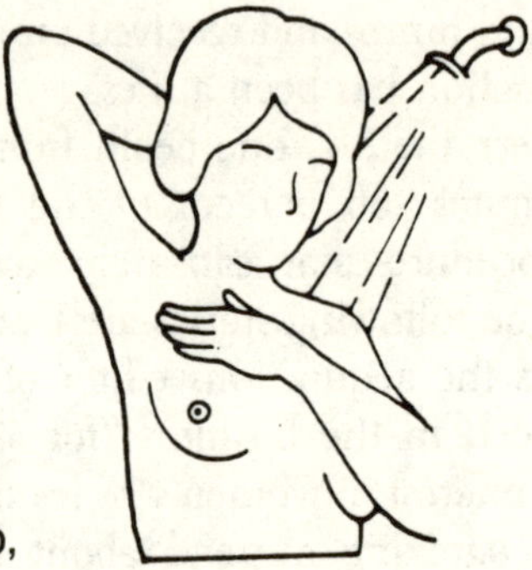

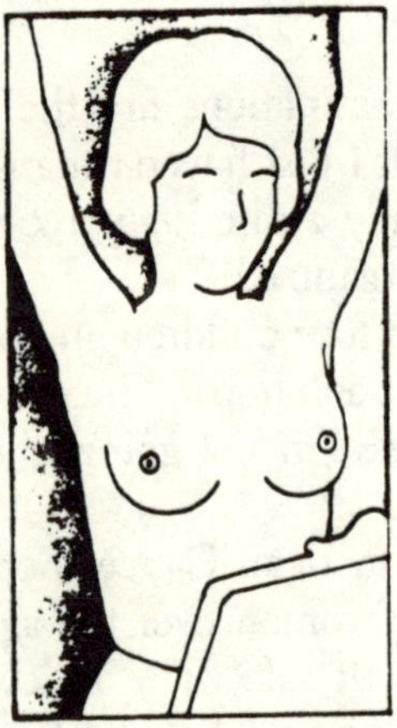

2 Before a mirror: Inspect your breasts with arms at your sides. Next, raise your arms high overhead. Look for any changes in contour of each breast, a swelling, dimpling of skin or changes in the nipple.

Then, rest palms on hips and press down firmly to flex your chest muscles. Left and right breasts will not exactly match—few women's breasts do.

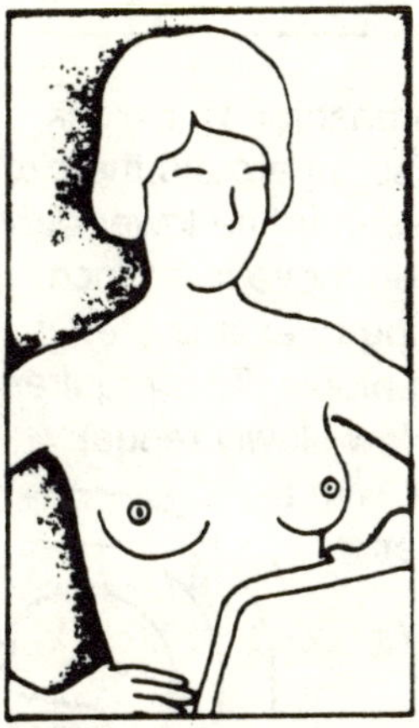

Regular inspection shows what is normal for you and will give you confidence in your examination.

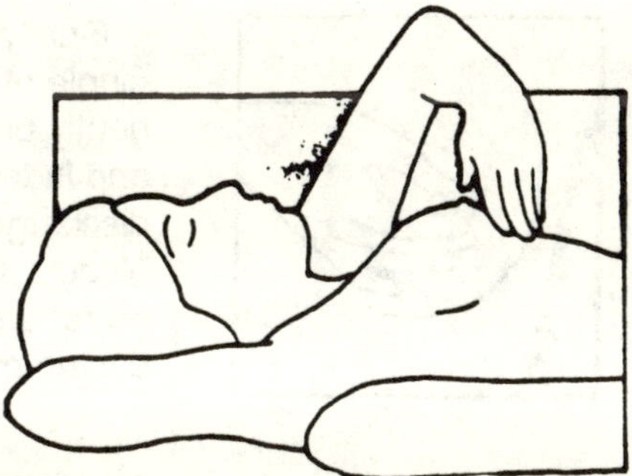

3 Lying down:
To examine your right breast, put a pillow or folded towel under your right shoulder. Place right hand behind your head—this distributes breast tissue more evenly on the chest. With left hand, fingers flat, press gently in small circular motions around an imaginary clock face. Begin at

outermost top of your right breast for 12 o'clock, then move to 1 o'clock, and so on around the circle back to 12. A ridge of firm tissue in the lower curve of each breast is normal. Then move in an inch, toward the nipple, keep circling to examine *every part of your breast,* including nipple. This requires at least three more circles. Now slowly repeat procedure on your left breast with a pillow under your left shoulder and left hand behind head. Notice how your breast structure feels.

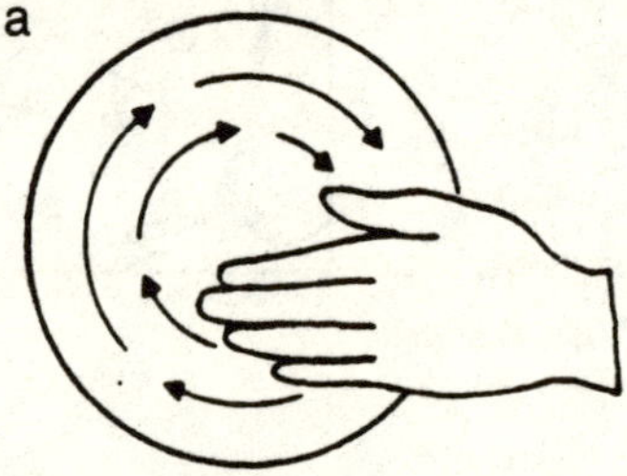

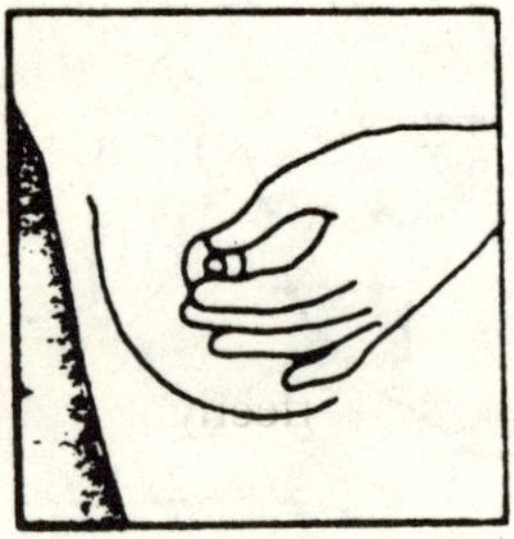

Finally, squeeze the nipple of each breast gently between thumb and index finger. Any discharge, clear or bloody, should be reported to your doctor immediately.

The National Cancer Institute report on breast cancer noted that women who are taught breast self-examination by a doctor are more likely to practice it than women who learn the technique in other ways. The next time you see your physician, even if you have been regularly examining your breasts, ask that he or she review the procedure with you.

Many women examining their breasts have said that they really do not know how they can tell the difference between a common lump and a cancerous one. It is difficult to distinguish between the two. Eight of ten lumps are benign. A cancerous lump is usually hard and solid. It is difficult to delineate. It does not move around if you touch it. It is usually painless. It is found most often in the outer quadrants of the breast. Other signs might include a skin dimpling over the tumor. Sometimes a nipple may be retracted, or it may discharge some fluid. The fluid may be clear, milky, or even tinged with blood and pus. When examining your breasts, look at the darker area around the nipple, the areola: If you can see a partial discoloration as if it were chapped, be certain to call your physician.

Become accustomed to looking at your breasts in front of a mirror, so that you can see changes just as they begin to occur. Do not be concerned, however, if one breast is larger than the other. That is common. Nature does not always make perfectly symmetrical people.

Is there any way to distinguish symptoms of a malignant tumor from symptoms of other breast diseases? Yes, but only with the help of a physician.

Other Detection Methods

Along with breast self-examination, the most successful of all detection methods is mammography, which is simply an x-ray of the breast. Some women have been afraid of mammography, thinking that radiation exposure itself caused cancer. That might have been true years ago, when women received seven or eight rads (units of absorbed radiation) every time they had a breast x-ray. Today the machines at modern facilities emit less than one rad.

When you have a mammogram, try to go to a major center where the radiologist's specialty is breasts. Dr. Marc Homer, chief of the Mammography Section of the Tufts-New England Medical Center, which has been funded to become a Breast Cancer Center for the northeastern United States, has said, "A small hospital center may do only two mammograms a week. A large hospital center such as Massachusetts General might do as many as sixty per day. Some women are put off by the large assembly-line notion. They should not be. With breast cancer detection, you want to use someone who is technically expert at taking a first rate x-ray and interpreting it as well. Also, some machines are more modern and more effective than other machines, with less radiation used."

When you go to the center for a mammogram, ask how many are done each day or each week. If you must travel to a larger center nearby, it is worth the trip.

There are a number of questions that come to mind before an initial mammography. What constitutes a baseline examination? Is a single film enough? Is the commonly used two-view technique, with two x-rays, a better screening technique? Should two films be taken one year apart to establish a basis for comparison?

At the moment there are no definite answers, although the Guttman Institute in New York City and other institutions are studying such questions.

Dr. Homer feels that when you are having your first set of x-rays, two views should be done. "Of course two views are better than one," he says. "We suggest just one for reasons of cost, but I would want my own wife to have two. I would especially suggest this if a woman is high risk. She should have two angles.

"All of these questions can only be answered on an individual basis, however. But women should not make the decision against two x-rays on the basis of their fear of excess radiation, because the exposure is miniscule," he declares.

While some women still have negative feelings about mammography, the fact is that in long-term studies, *its effectiveness as a detection method is unparalleled*. In a report by the American Cancer Society, Dr. Henry Leis noted that the ten-year survival rate for patients with breast cancer of less than one centimeter in size (about the size of a large pea) diagnosed by mammography was 97.1. And according to Dr. Philip Strax of the Guttman Institute, major studies show that substantial numbers of cancers detected by radiation could *not* have been detected by any other means.

The American Cancer Society has issued the following recommendations for breast examinations:

Type of Examination	*Age*	*Frequency of Examination*
Breast self-examination	Over 20	Every month
Physical examination by physician	20–40	Every three years
	Over 40	Every Year
Mammography	Under 35	Only if symptoms appear
	35–40	Baseline should be established
	40–50	Consult personal physician
	Over 50	Every year

Besides mammography, other tests also are being used, but they are much less precise. These tests include:

Alcohol sponge test In this test, developed by Drs. Henry Leis and Maurice Black, an alcohol-soaked sponge is used to wet the breast. In women with breast cancer, the skin over the tumor shows a discreet blush that appears for a few minutes, then starts to fade.

Thermography More heat emanates from some tumors than from normal-tissue working cells. A sophisticated machine renders the most minute temperature variations and heat emissions as multicolored patterns. This method appears to be perfectly safe—no radiation is used—but results are not always dependable. Sometimes a noncancerous tumor looks like a malignant one, and a malignant tumor might even go undetected because the circulatory system is not bringing sufficient blood to the area to bring about an increase in heat. For this test, you spend about fifteen minutes in a cooled room, nude from the waist up with your arms raised slightly. (Touching the skin with the arms can create enough friction to raise the body temperature.)

Xeroradiography This technique is similar to mammography. The image of the breast, however, is produced on a special coated paper, not on x-ray film. It probably is as accurate as mammography, though it is less generally available.

Graphic stress telethermography Placing your hands in ice water will lower your body temperature. In this test, after the body temperature is lowered, the breasts are examined. Warm spots may indicate tumors. The test is not sufficiently accurate.

Sonography In recent years, the use of ultrasound has been hailed as a significant advance in medical technology. Many pregnant women now have ultrasound tests to determine their baby's size and position. High-frequency sound waves are sent into the body through a small device that looks like a microphone. The waves bounce back and are translated into an image on a screen. The method shows promise, but is not yet proven in breast cancer detection.

Biopsy The surest means of diagnosis for breast cancer, a biopsy involves the surgical removal of a piece of tissue from the breast or the removal of the entire growth if it is tiny enough. Once this is done, the tissue can be analyzed microscopically for cancer cells. A biopsy for detecting breast cancer differs from a needle aspiration, in which fluid is drawn from a cyst. The needle technique is used when the physician thinks that a swelling is probably a nonmalignant cyst.

The American Cancer Society notes that about 80 percent of all breast lumps biopsied are benign. The biopsy procedure itself, however, has been a cause of controversy. Until 1979, when the National Cancer Institute issued new guidelines concerning treatment of breast cancer, biopsies were done under anesthesia in a hospital. If you had a biopsy, a section would be immediately analyzed, while you were in the operating room, and if malignancy were present, the breast would be removed right away. In a frozen section the lump is quick-frozen, sliced thinly, and viewed (after staining) through a microscope. The whole procedure takes less than twenty minutes.

Largely through the efforts of Rose Kushner of the Women's Breast Cancer Advisory Center, Inc., this practice is fading. It had two distinct disadvantages. The "frozen section," as this type of biopsy was called, was not always accurate. In addition, hundreds of women faced the prospect of being ushered into an operating room not knowing whether they would emerge with one breast or two. *The New England Journal of Medicine,* reporting on the proceedings of a Consensus Development Conference in 1979, said that a two-step procedure should be done in most cases.

Today there are two recommended biopsy options. You may choose to see a physician who will do the biopsy in his or her office under local anesthesia, or you may go to a minor surgery room at a hospital where you will be given anesthesia. The biopsy will be done, and after a few hours, you will be permitted to return home. A laboratory will take twenty-four to seventy-two hours to analyze the biopsy.

If you are scheduled for a biopsy, make certain that your surgeon also has made arrangements for an estrogen receptor assay. The preparations for the assay must be done *immediately* after the tumor is removed. Some tumors are estrogen-dependent and others estrogen-independent. The information from the assay can help the physician determine the course of your treatment. An estrogen-dependent breast tumor is one that reacts to estrogens manufactured by the ovaries. In the early 1940s and 50s, because there was some belief that ovarian hormones played a role in breast cancer, when women had mastectomies, surgeons immediately removed the ovaries as well in some cases. This is no longer done. However, if a tumor is estrogen-dependent, your physician might consider hormone manipulation. Hormonal manipulation is accomplished in several ways. It might include removal of functioning estrogen-producing ovaries, which is done generally in younger women, and may lead to better control of certain breast cancers. Curiously in older patients, the administration of estrogen may improve the patient's condition. There are drugs which interfere with the action of estrogen and these may be useful. To control widespread disease, removal of the adrenal or pituitary glands may reduce body hormone production and offer temporary help.

If the tumor is estrogen-*in*dependent, you may receive chemotherapy.

WHAT IF THE DIAGNOSIS IS CANCER?

A diagnosis of breast cancer means that there is a nodule of malignant cells in your breast. Cancer spreads via the lymph system to the lymph nodes in the armpit. It may also spread to the lymph nodes behind the breastbone, to the neck over the collarbone. Untreated, this cancer can spread to the bone, liver, lungs, and brain. Breast cancer is an extremely complex disease. It is believed that there are at least fifteen different types ranging from slow- to fast-growing.

If you are told that you have cancer of the breast, you should ask your physician which type of cancer he or she suspects. You might also get a second opinion from a pathologist as well as another physician. You will want to know what treatment choices exist, since these vary according to how far the cancer has advanced. Physicians describe four different stages.

Stage O and Stage I

The earliest detectable stage of breast cancer (Stage O) is called carcinoma *in situ*. It is believed to be equivalent to the completely curable cancer precursors found in the endometrium and the cervix. The deposits of cells in this type of early cancer generally are so small that even a physician probably could not feel them, so carcinoma *in situ* of the breast may be detected most often through mammography. This stage is almost always curable. Sometimes a simple biopsy, which is usually considered a diagnostic tool, might be sufficient treatment for removing the entire cancer at this very early stage.

While local treatment might be sufficient, it is still possible that even at the early stage, breast removal will be necessary. In the United States, mastectomies have been the preferred treatment for any type of breast cancer. What is important to remember, however, is that in the treatment of early breast cancer options do exist. Options for the *in situ* stage of breast cancer are the same as those for Stage I of the disease.

Stage I usually refers to tumors that can be *felt* but are still quite small, that is, less than two centimeters in diameter (about the size of a large pea). The prognosis is good and local treatment should be sufficient.

Local treatments can include the simple biopsy we discussed above, radiation therapy, and possibly a local excision—called a lumpectomy—to remove the tumor. More drastically, a simple mastectomy might also be required.

On July 2, 1981, *The New England Journal of Medicine* reported that minimal treatment for breast cancer seems sufficient when the tumor is less than two centimeters, and without palpable lymph node involvement. According to the authors of the article, mastectomies "appear to involve unnecessary mutilation!"

Radiation treatment alone is being advocated for the very earliest cases of breast disease, when the tumor is less than two centimeters and physicians do not feel it has spread to the adjacent lymph nodes. This is not a new procedure. It was done as far back as the early 1930s when Sir Geoffrey Keynes developed a technique to remove the primary tumor and then implant radium needles in the breast and nearby regions.

As the procedure is done today, radioactive material in tiny containers is implanted in the patient's breast while she is under anesthesia. The radioactive implant remains in the breast for two or three days and then is removed, generally with no side effects other than mild local discomfort. External radiation from a cobalt 60 machine or equivalent can be used.

At the National Cancer Institute Breast Cancer Conference in 1979, Dr. Samuel Hellman of the Harvard Medical School reported on 136 patients who were treated there with such implants—tiny containers of radioactive material. He found that 91 percent of the women survived for five years. This is comparable to the survival rate for women receiving mastectomies at this early stage. At the present time, radiation treatment is being used in very select—very early—cases.

Some physicians fear the radium in one breast may have unwanted side effects on a younger woman's other breast. Because the procedure has been used for less than twenty years, long-term follow-up studies are not available. The reports from NCI, however, were encouraging. You should investigate this option if you find a very early cancer.

Simple Mastectomy

In the early stages (I and II), the simple mastectomy with

radiation may be the preferred treatment. This depends on your physician and your own ability to make an intelligent choice. In simple mastectomy, only the breast is removed; no muscles or underlying tissue are cut away. A simple mastectomy is generally planned if the surgeon believes that the tumor is early, small, and has not spread to the nodes. If the nearby nodes are, indeed, found to be involved with cancer at the time of surgery, radiation can be added. Many physicians feel that this is equally effective as the more radical procedures that remove underlying muscle tissue and take out all the nodes in the axilla (armpit). Even for somewhat more advanced tumors, the simple mastectomy plus radiation seems to be just as effective as the more radical procedures in some ongoing studies.

Stage II

Stage II cancer refers to tumors between two and five centimeters in diameter. The cancer at this stage may have spread to the lymph nodes within the breast but not to other organs. Since at this stage it is suspected that the lymph nodes are involved, simple mastectomy (which involves only the removal of the breast) is not usually the treatment of choice. It is at this stage of cancer that treatment choices can be most controversial. The possibilities range from a local excision, as discussed in connection with Stage I cancer, if the tumor is less than three inches in diameter to complete removal of the breast and the underlying muscles.

Full-scale surgery—as opposed to local excision—is to be expected in most cases. This is the treatment of choice. The controversies revolve around the question of *how much* surgery is necessary, not about the need for surgery itself. The two main choices that you and your doctor must consider are:

The standard radical mastectomy (also called the Halsted mastectomy) In this operation, the entire breast is removed, along with the underlying pectoral muscles and much of the adjacent armpit, including the fat and lymph glands. This operation is extensive and disfiguring. It makes breast reconstruction very difficult, but not impossible. For many years, starting in 1948, this operation was the standard way of treating breast cancer. Many conservative physicians still believe it offers the best chance of a cure. By removing more flesh, they feel they have a better chance of getting rid of all the cancer cells.

The modified radical mastectomy (MRM) This operation is newer and somewhat less drastic than the standard radical mastectomy. The entire breast is removed, along with the lymph glands in the armpit. The pectoral muscles are left intact, however, thus greatly facilitating breast reconstruction later on. The patient also will heal more quickly after an MRM.

Is this less drastic operation as effective as the other? The answers are still coming in, but so far they are encouraging.

In a 1979 report on a five-year follow-up study of 1,680 women, Dr. Bernard Fischer, coordinator of the National Surgical Adjuvant Breast Project, said there was no difference in the survival rates between women who underwent standard radical mastectomies and those who had modified radical mastectomies.

Whichever form the surgery takes, the physician may suggest follow-up radiation treatments. These would be external radiation treatments, not the radiation implants used to treat Stage I breast cancer. Depending on the nature of the cancer, you might also go on to chemotherapy; this treatment is discussed in Chapter 11.

Stage III

Stage III means that the tumor is greater than five centimeters (about two inches in diameter) and probably has spread to the lymph nodes. This does not necessarily mean the cancer has spread to other organs, although it is a possibility. A conservative surgeon might suggest the standard radical mastectomy at this stage. Make

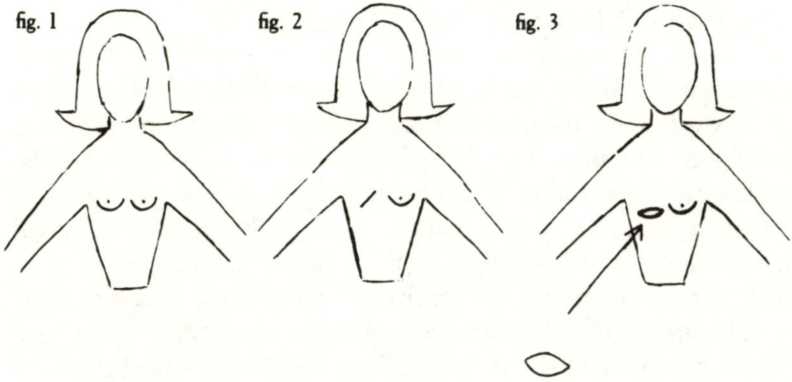

BREAST RECONSTRUCTION

Fig. 1. Breasts before mastectomy. Fig. 2. The incision site. At this time most physicians will attempt to determine the best method for future reconstruction, if possible or if discussed in advance with a woman. Fig. 3. A pocket will be made in the chest region to accomodate an implant which is then inserted to create a breast mound.

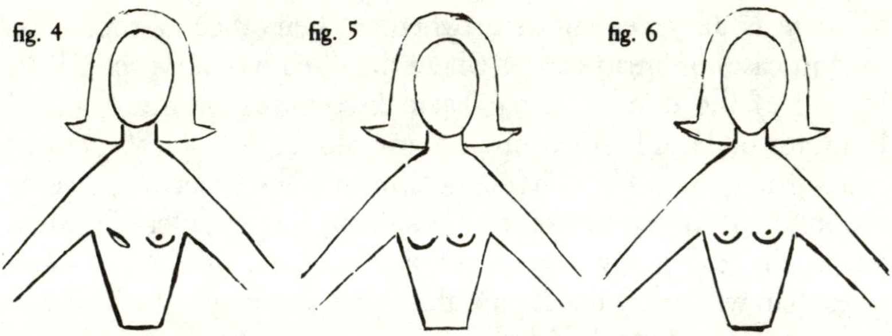

Fig. 4. When more extensive surgery had been performed on an original mastectomy, a skin flap is created and then the implant is inserted. This is a longer, more complex type of surgery. Fig. 5. The breast mound is created without a nipple in most cases. The wound is closed and sutured. Fig. 6. The nipple reconstruction is the last procedure. It can be recreated in a number of ways; sometimes the nipple from the breast removed will be preserved and regrafted.

certain that you believe this to be necessary. Get a second opinion. It is possible that the modified radical mastectomy would be just as effective. In either case, surgery at this stage usually will be followed by chemotherapy and/or radiation. It may be that you will have to make a trade—that is, having the modified radical mastectomy, which is the less drastic of the two operations, *may* mean you will need more intensive chemotherapy and/or radiation.

The use of chemotherapy has become another controversial issue in the treatment of breast cancer. Favorable results have been cited by Dr. James Holland of the Mount Sinai School of Medicine in New York City, with combination treatments that usually include cytoxan, methotrexate, and 5-FU. In addition, a study conducted in Milan under the auspices of the National Cancer Institute of Italy and reported by Dr. Gianni Bonadonna indicated that in patients whose breast cancer had already spread, the survival rate was substantially and significantly increased by the use of combination drugs following surgery.

There is disagreement as to whether chemotherapy should be used in cases of breast cancer where the disease has not spread. In Stage I of the disease, it has been discouraged by the National Institutes of Health since mastectomy alone gives an 80 percent survival rate. Wouldn't chemotherapy help the other 20 percent? Possibly, but to give everyone chemotherapy as a matter of routine means that too many women receive too much toxicity in more cases than will be useful. Again, this is a question about which you should seek individual advice.

Stage IV

This stage is called metastatic. The tumor cells have spread (metastisized) throughout the body. The outlook for long-term survival is not good. There are methods, however, of prolonging life and relieving pain.

Physicians are working with certain forms of immunotherapy in attempting to bring relief to women with this stage of cancer. A drug released on the market in 1979. tamoxifen citrate, which can be taken in pill form, has been useful in bringing about pain relief with certain types of metastatic breast cancer.

Experimental treatments also are being offered in some programs for patients who appear to have incurable cancer. Ask your physician whether such a program exists in your area and whether you qualify. There also are many breast cancer study groups in the United States today. Some study groups accept women no matter what the stage of their cancer. If you find yourself at this stage of the disease, it is worth investigating.

WHAT IS THE PROGNOSIS WHEN THE DIAGNOSIS IS BREAST CANCER?

The American Cancer Society in *Cancer Statistics, 1981* reports an 85 percent cure rate when breast cancer is detected early. When it has regionalised, that is, spread, but not necessarily to distant sites, the survival rates drop to 56 percent. Metastases are cancer, spread to very distant sites. It also noted that only 48 percent of the cases of breast cancer were detected at the localized stage; in 41 percent of the cases the cancer had already spread. In other words, half the women who develop breast cancer are not getting optimal treatment because their cancer is not detected soon enough.

EMOTIONAL SIDE EFFECTS OF CANCER

Geraldine and her husband were both college professors who lived on a tiny estate in the Vermont countryside. They considered themselves down-to-earth people who could accept whatever life had to offer, "no matter how the cards are dealt to us."

Then one day Geraldine went in for a check-up, "the first I had had in a hundred years," and was told she had breast cancer. "This was really a time to reevaluate my life and my relationships." For two weeks Geraldine sulked and said nothing. When she broke the news to her husband, he fell apart.

"After the surgery, I went into a terrible depression thinking our sex life would be over. I started talking to the other women in town and they told me all the horror stories about the nearby women whose husbands went off and found themselves younger women. I just knew it was going to happen to my marriage.

"The depression was so bad that I had to take a longer leave of absence from the college than I had anticipated. When I finally got up the courage to go back and teach, every time I looked at one of my full-breasted students, I cried. Suddenly, I became a pill taker. For about two months, my relationship with my husband was terrible. Then finally one night he said, 'Geraldine, let's talk about it.' We expressed our feelings and went for counseling, and our marriage is better than ever."

In *A Crisis to Grow On* by Roberta Klein, a medical social worker asked, "How many husbands, guilty of their inability to help the patient, resign themselves to vitiated and often destructive marriages? How many children develop school problems in response to an unexplained and mysterious depression in their mothers?

"Patients are often aided and abetted in their inability to deal with the crisis of losing a breast by family who are either insensitive to patients' cues or . . . find the problem equally painful to face," says Ms. Klein. "For the mastectomy patient to return to equilibrium, she must accept the loss of her breast by fully mourning for that loss. This necessarily includes grief around the fears that she might lose her husband or even ultimately her life, and she must reintegrate her self-image as worthy of love and the rewards of life."

How can other people help? They can encourage her to express her feelings and help her sort out the real from the unreal terrors. If her doctor has not already done so, he can refer her to the American Cancer Society's Reach to Recovery volunteers, all of whom have undergone this surgery. It is most important for a woman to feel loved and wanted after this type of surgery.

Many of the books written by women and for women that deal with the emotional side effects of breast cancer also can be comforting. Those who have lost a breast and have related their feelings in books include the news correspondent Betty Rollin, former First Lady Betty Ford, and actress Ingrid Bergman. Susan Sontag also had breast cancer. In her book *Illness As Metaphor*, she discusses not breast cancer but the concept of the disease. Many women have said that Ms. Sontag seems to capture just why it is that even today some women shy away from admitting they have had cancer.

THE RECONSTRUCTION OPTION

Janice was just thirty when she learned she had breast cancer. Since her mother had had the disease, she was well aware that she herself was a high-risk person. She had discussed all the options of treatment with her physician even before she discovered the lump in her breast. Because she had seen how much difficulty her mother had had adjusting to wearing a prosthesis, Janice made the immediate choice for reconstructive surgery.

But there are no physical reasons for making the choice right away. This is a decision that can be deferred until you are comfortable with it.

Evan, for instance, managed a busy New England restaurant. She struggled with a prosthesis for more than fifteen years after a radical mastectomy, then decided to investigate the possibility of reconstruction. She was delighted to learn that she would not only receive a new breast but have her other breast balanced to match.

A reconstruction may involve one or more operations to recreate the shape of a woman's lost breast. There are a number of different procedures for reconstruction, but basically the idea is to form a pocket into which a package of silicone gel is placed. If too much skin was removed in the initial mastectomy, a skin flap might have to be created. In addition, nipples can be made using tissue from the vaginal area or tissue saved from the original breast (the "banked" nipple).

Usually women with Stage II cancer are candidates for reconstruction. If you have cancer that is in Stage I you might consider either radiation implants or a simple lumpectomy. Dr. Marc Homer notes that if you are a twenty-five-year-old with Stage I cancer, you might consider having a mastectomy and reconstruction. Why? "Because no long-term studies have been done to determine the effect of the radiation implants alone and how they might affect the other breast. In general, surgeons agree that Stage II women can safely consider reconstruction," Dr. Homer says.

If you have Stage II, this means that the cancer may have spread and the prognosis is less positive. Stage IV indicates metastases, and reconstruction should not be a consideration.

Women of any age can have reconstruction. Most surgeons only suggest it for their "young patients," however, and many seem to feel that women in their fifites are—or should be—less concerned about their appearance. Too often the attitude has been, "Why do you want reconstruction? You should be happy just to be alive." Dr. Philip Corso disagrees with this advice. A clinical instructor in plastic surgery at Yale University School of Medicine, he feels that any woman who wishes reconstruction should have it. His oldest "reconstructed" patient was seventy-four years old, and he said she "thinks like a thirty-five-year old . . . whose positive attitude will help her outlive us all!"

While reconstruction may be discouraged if there is a suspicion that a woman may not live more than five years, some doctors have wondered whether this attitude does not "nail the coffin." One physician said, "I discouraged reconstruction in a woman who I felt couldn't live for more than three years. Then I realized, 'What if I'm wrong, and she does live?' If I'm right and she doesn't live, would reconstruction have made her happier? In either case, who was I to discourage her?"

Physicians are finally coming to see what many women have been saying all along: Reconstruction adds to a woman's positive feelings about herself. Some women can learn to live without a breast and without experiencing permanent emotional trauma. Other women cannot. Some women will not let their husbands touch them, or see them undressed, after they have lost a breast. Some women refuse to look at their own bodies and will dress and undress in closets. Some women want reconstruction because they feel that they will have better sex lives with their husbands or lovers.

The reasons for which reconstruction is chosen do not matter. You should not have to make excuses for this choice. If you want reconstruction, investigate the possibility.

The cost of reconstruction can be very high, up to $10,000. Most medical plans today have insurance coverage for the surgery. A typical hospital bill of $7,000 might be completely covered and cost you no more than $10—for phone calls from the hospital.

Reconstruction Procedures

If you want reconstruction, the time to speak up is before a mastectomy. In the past so many women got hostile reactions from their surgeons that they became discouraged. Part of the physicians' negative attitude stemmed from the fact that the state of the art of reconstruction ten years ago was not nearly so advanced as it now is. Today reconstructed breasts can be quite natural-looking.

If you discuss reconstruction beforehand with your surgeon, he or she will most likely send you to a plastic surgeon to discuss the surgery. Although the reconstruction will not take place immediately, the surgeon may ask the plastic surgeon to do the initial incision at the time of the mastectomy. Sometimes a surgeon sympathetic with the wishes for reconstruction will have a rapport with a plastic surgeon and learn just what type of incision to make. Also plans will be made to save the nipple, if possible.

Not until you have completed radiation and chemotherapy treatments, if these are required, will the actual reconstructive surgery take place. Usually, you also have to wait until the mastectomy is healed—between three months and one year.

Not all plastic surgeons are equally skilled in all reconstruction techniques, and the technique that will be best for you depends upon the kind of mastectomy you had. So how can you determine which surgeon and which technique is right for you?

There appear to be few standard approaches to reconstructive breast surgery; there may be several approaches which are variations on a theme. Basically breast reconstruction includes the placement of a prosthesis (silicons or other material gel) shaped like the inner part of the breast, inside of a pocket made in the breast.

If you have had the classical radical mastectomy (the Halsted type), it is often necessary to have a type of surgery called the myocutaneous flap, or latissimus dorsi flap. This is usually a procedure in which skin and muscle tissues are rotated from the back to cover the mastectomy area. It can often be a one-step procedure, but it may take many hours and it carries with it some risk of infection. It is important that you find a surgeon experienced in this technique. How many operations does the good plastic surgeon perform? That is a difficult question to answer. Although there are about 100,000 mastectomies performed each year, only 1 to 5 percent of all women have reconstruction. Yet there are experts in the field who have been doing the surgery for a number of years. One of these physicians is Dr. Saul Hoffman of the Mount Sinai School of Medicine.

Dr. Hoffman feels that most reconstructive surgery is safe and effective. "It is important, however, for women to realize just what to expect. There are limitations to reconstruction, but once a woman realizes what these limitations are, she is usually very satisfied," he said.

The limitation on reconstruction lies in the inability of any surgeon to perfectly duplicate an actual breast. The few pioneers tend to be in great demand, and some women have been put off by the assembly-line atmosphere in some of their offices.

Helen LaGatutta, of Rye, New York, decided upon reconstruction after fourteen years of living with a prosthesis. She took the time to interview physicians, talk to other women who had reconstruction, and asked to see pictures—not just from the surgeons' own files, but from other women as well. Presently working to set up a chapter for women seeking advice on reconstruction, she said, "With enough phone calls, you can find surgeons locally who have the expertise and the time to spend with you to make you feel comfortable about the reconstructive surgery."

There has been a great deal of controversy concerning reconstruction procedures. Arthur Holleb, chief medical officer of the American Cancer Society, advises that you have a working partnership with a surgeon whom you trust, so that he or she might help you make the decision as to which type of plastic surgery technique is best for you.

A New York-based organization called AFTER (see Appendix C), for Ask a Friend to Explain Reconstruction, has this advice:

• Ask to talk to and see other women who have had reconstructive surgery.

• Understand that there are different procedures and different types of implants. There are advantages and disadvantages to procedures and implants alike. Examine the implants carefully.

• Ask the surgeon how many reconstructions he or she has done.

• Ask to see pictures. (Some surgeons do not show pictures, but they will give you a list of names of women whom they have reconstructed who will talk to you and show you the results of their own surgery.)

CAUSES AND PREVENTION OF BREAST CANCER

It is simple enough to state that researchers believe that breast cancer might be linked to diet, viruses, environmental factors, or a woman's estrogen system. There are studies that point to any and all of these factors; breast cancer is a disease of controversy.

Today, however, the link between diet and breast cancer is so strong that the National Cancer Institute issued a formal statement in 1979 on diet, nutrition, and cancer. What the Institute and other researchers have found is that the dietary link may consist not so much of carcinogens or polluted food or water but rather of the Western world's tendency to overnutrition. In those countries where fatty meat is not the main source of protein, breast cancer rates drop significantly. Japanese women have a low breast cancer rate; in 1981, figures reported from 1974-1975 studies indicated that only 4.8 of every 100,000 women in Japan died of the disease. In Thailand, deaths from breast cancer number 1.1 in 100,000. Look at the chart below: The dietary fat intake of the Japanese is about forty grams per day. By contrast, in the United States, where 22.1 of every 100,000 women died of breast cancer in 1980, the fat intake per day ranges from 140 to 160 grams. (Because of reporting methods, these figures are considered current.)

The National Cancer Institute report also says that "fats are known to change the metabolism of many tissues in humans, possibly affecting the relation of various hormones to tissue growth. The case for this is strongest for *breast cancer*, where hormonal environment has been shown to influence the susceptibility of cancer."

DIETARY FAT IN RELATION TO TUMOR DEVELOPMENT

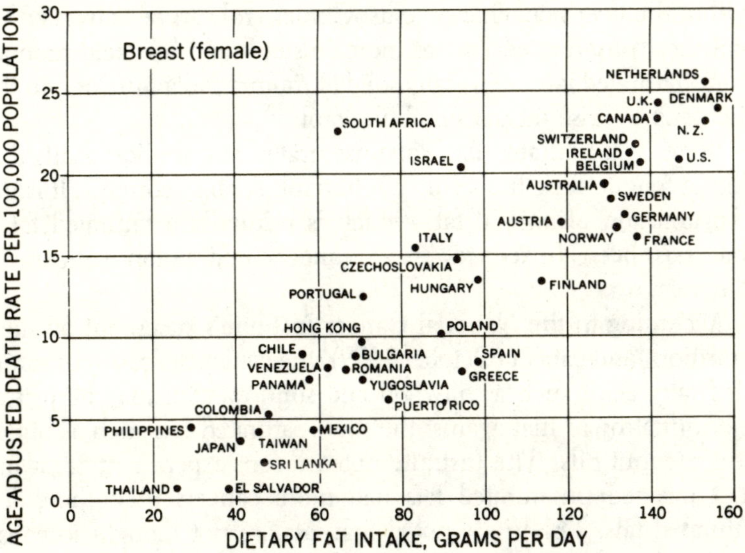

From *Malignant Neglect*, by Environmental Defense Fund and Robert H. Boyle. Copyright © 1979 by Environmental Defense Fund and Robert H. Boyle. Reprinted by permission of Alfred A. Knopf, Inc.

Why is it that in third-world countries breast cancer is rare while in industrialized societies—the United States, Canada, and Western Europe—it is rampant? Researchers are suggesting that our fat content "alters the body's balance of sex hormones, which in some as yet undetermined way increases susceptibility to breast cancer."

Dr. Joseph J. Vitale, a nutrition-pathologist who is associate dean for International Health at the Boston University School of Medicine, noted that the food we eat can affect us in several different ways. For example, foods can:

• promote absorptive properties of the tissues.

• carry possible carcinogens or promote change in intestinal bacteria so that carcinogenises (cancer production) is made easier.

• modify our defense mechanisms so that we cannot defend ourselves against carcinogenesis.

Some foods that we eat may be turned into carcinogenic agents within the liver's enzyme systems. Cholesterol can be converted, as can most unsaturated fats, to increase sterol and bile acid production. Saturated fats are usually solid at room temperature and in the diet tend to raise the serum cholesterol.

Butter is a saturated fat. Polyunsaturated fats are liquid oils that do not tend to raise the serum cholesterol, such as corn oil. It is the consumption of animal fat—which is primarily a saturated fat—that has been linked to breast cancers and colon cancers in America.

According to the National Cancer Institute's statement on diet, nutrition, and cancer (October 1979), the evidence against unsaturated fatty acids such as olive oil and sunflower oil may be just as incriminating as that against the more saturated fats such as butter and coconut oils. The Institute noted recent experiments showing that rats fed unsaturated fats had more cancers than those fed saturated fats. Dr. Vitale noted that fats are not thought to cause cancer directly but to somehow influence metabolic processes of normal cells to make them more susceptible to the development of cancer caused by other agents.

Dr. Ernest Wynder of the American Health Association has long been advocating a more prudent diet. "We know the lower-fat diets have been beneficial in heart patients and we have strong evidence that they will help prevent more increases in cancer," he said.

If fat is indeed a contributing cause of breast cancer, then to alter your diet would be a means of prevention. In addition, you might want to begin seriously looking at your overall diet in terms of nutritional requirements.

There are theories that breast cancer can be prevented with a balance of nutritional foods and vitamin supplements. Carlton Fredericks, the well-known nutritionist, has written *Breast Cancer: A Nutritional Approach*. While this nutritional approach to prevention has not been proven to be effective, few will argue that a woman eating a nutritionally balanced diet low in fats will probably feel healthier and be healthier. She *may* also be reducing her cancer risk. Some theories claim that estriol/estrone plus estradiol ratio plays a role in breast cancer prevention; this ratio can be manipulated through the diet. Dr. Fredericks points to the diets of the Japanese and the Chinese in their native countries as helping to control the disease.

In terms of cancer prevention, some have suspected that breast feeding a child may protect women in some way. The protective mechanism of breast feeding was a popular theory until a carefully controlled study conducted by Brian McMahon of the Harvard University School of Public Health found no appreciable differences in the breast-feeding history among patients with and without breast cancer. Many people, however, point to the story of the boat people of Hong Kong. The Tonka women in Hong Kong only nurse their babies with their right breast. When breast cancer is found in these women, it is in the left breast. This study was reported in *The Lancet*, a well-known British journal of medicine.

Another interesting idea concerns the possible release of substances from the brain such as chemicals that control the pituitary when the nipples are stimulated in sex play. It has been suggested that these substances may lessen the risk of subsequent breast cancer, but this idea has not been proven.

Theories that viruses cause human breast cancer also remain unproven. The Special Report of November 20, 1980, in *The New England Journal of Medicine* states: "There is no good evidence that a virus transmitted from one case to another has a role in human breast cancer. A virus transmitted from parent to offspring and integrated with the genome [gene] may still be identified, but it is difficult to see what preventive action could follow from such information." But in certain *mice*, breast cancer virus is transmitted from mother to daughter by nursing.

Environmental factors involved in breast cancer were reported in women who were treated with multiple fluoroscopies for pulmonary tuberculosis who had an increase in breast cancer. There also was an increased incidence of breast cancer among survivors of the atomic bomb. Today it is suggested that women avoid excessive radiation to the breast. Do keep in mind that the amount of radiation received from a mammography, which is usually just under one rad, is only two to three times greater than you receive from a normal chest x-ray.

Perhaps the newest, most controversial means of preventing breast cancer is the prophylactic subcutaneous mastectomy, that is, breast removal in high-risk women even *before* a cancer is detected. Some doctors suggest that a woman who has cancer in one breast, because she faces an increased risk of developing cancer in the second breast, should have the additional surgery, particularly if she is in her twenties or thirties. Still other doctors oppose the idea of prophylactic surgery completely.

With detection methods and minimal treatments so readily available for women in whom cancer is detected early, and with a prognosis of a nearly 90 percent chance of survival when the cancer is found early, if you are considering breast removal for prevention, ask yourself, "Why?" Be certain to have at least two opinions. Be certain you understand that any and all surgery, no matter how simple, carries risks. Do be aware, however, that there is a five times greater chance of developing cancer in the remaining breast.

REMINDERS

If you know you are at high risk for breast cancer, on your next office visit discuss options with your physician; later, if you are in a panic situation, you might not make the best choices.

Find out now where you will be treated if you should ever need to have a lump biopsied—would you go to a local hospital or a major cancer center? Would you use your own physician or would you seek the help of a specialist? Since the American College of Surgeons says that general surgeons do approximately ten mastectomies a year, you might feel more comfortable with a breast cancer specialist who does several mastectomies each month. Discuss in advance with your physician your options for having the biopsy done as a separate procedure. It is your right, and you should not give consent to simultaneous surgery unless, after discussion with your physician, *you* are convinced that this is the best course of action for you.

What about a second opinion? It is perhaps most valuable to seek the second opinion of a pathologist rather than a surgeon, particularly if there is doubt about the first set of findings. If you do have a mastectomy, ask to have a Reach to Recovery volunteer visit you when the surgery is over.

If you are considering reconstruction, find a surgeon who might be able to help you take immediate steps to begin the reconstructive procedure. Contact AFTER. Find out whatever *new* information is available. If you really want the latest information on breast cancer, ask a librarian at your physician's hospital to help.

After examining all your options, sit down with your physician and ask his or her help in making the choice that is best for you. Then consult the doctor within you. Once your choice is made, *live with it*. Don't waste one minute of your time saying, "If only."

RECOMMENDED BOOKS

Breast Cancer, A Health Resource Guide. The National Women's Health Network, Washington, D.C., 1981.

"Breast Reconstruction," a pamphlet prepared by the National Association of Plastic Surgeons and distributed by the American Cancer Society.

Cope, Oliver, M.D. *The Breast: Its Problems, Benign and*

Malignant, and How to Deal with Them. Boston: Houghton Mifflin, 1977.

Crile, George, M.D. *What Women Should Know About the Breast Cancer Controversy.* New York: Pocket Books, 1974.

Fredericks, Carlton. *Breast Cancer: A Nutritional Approach.* New York: Grosset and Dunlap, 1977.

Kushner, Rose. *Why Me: What Every Woman Needs to Know About Breast Cancer To Save Her Life.* New York: Holt, Rinehart and Winston, 1981.

Rollin, Betty. *First You Cry.* New York: Signet, 1977.

RECOMMENDED ARTICLES

Brinton LA et al. Menopausal estrogen use and risk of breast cancer. *Cancer* 47:2517–22.

Canellos GP. The management of early breast cancer. *The New England Journal of Medicine* 306:1430–32.

Ernster VL et al. Effects of caffeine-free diet on benign breast disease: a randomized trial. *Surgery* 91:263–7.

Graham S et al. Diet in the epidemiology of breast cancer. *American Journal of Epidemiology* 116:68–75.

Kelsey JL et al. Exogenous estrogens and other factors in the epidemiology of breast cancer. *Journal of the National Cancer Institute* 67:327–33.

Kinne DW et al. Estrogen receptor protein in breast cancer as a predictor of recurrence. *Cancer* 47:2364–7.

Korcok M. Tamoxifen encouraging for breast cancer (news). *Journal of the American Medical Association.* 246:1872

Chapter Seven

The Ovaries and the Fallopian Tubes

Joan is in her mid-fifties, but she can easily pass for thirty-five. She is an energetic woman concerned about her health, appearance, and mental attitude. One of her favorite expressions, is, "When I die at 103, I want people to remember me as an outgoing, positive person."

When Joan was fifty-three, she began menopause. At fifty-four her periods stopped altogether. Then about a year and a half later she noticed that she was beginning to bleed just slightly. This occurred several times over the course of a month. Not one to play games with her health, Joan went to her gynecologist. With the bleeding she described, he suspected she might have endometrial cancer, and he suggested an immediate D and C.

During the surgical procedure, Joan's physician felt an enlarged ovary. Because the ovaries of menopausal women usually shrink, an enlargement often indicates a serious condition. The physician sent the tissue samples to be analyzed by a pathologist, but even before receiving the report, he realized that in Joan's case it would be best if she consented to further exploratory surgery.

The next day he discussed Joan's condition with her. He explained that tissue sample analysis showed she did not have endometrial or cervical cancer, but that the enlarged ovary could well be a sign of ovarian cancer. Joan decided against further surgery and left the hospital.

One week later, Joan returned to her gynecologist. "I've done some thinking. I really didn't feel I could reach an 'on the spot' decision in the hospital. Once I was home, in my own bed, in my own house, I really thought I might wait a few months to see if the ovary got smaller. But it worried me. I called an old family friend for a second opinion. He totally supported the idea of exploratory surgery, and I'm ready."

The definitive diagnosis for ovarian cancer can usually be made only at the time of surgery. Joan understood fully that a surgeon would not operate twice (once to make a diagnosis, and then later to operate) due to the inherent dangers of abdominal surgery and that she might discover after the operation that her ovaries were diseased and had to be removed. (This situation differs from breast surgery in which a biopsy can first be made.) In Joan's case, ovarian cancer was discovered and it had spread to the upper part of her abdomen. The surgeon was able to remove all the visible tumor. Later Joan was started on a course of chemotherapy with an experimental drug. Today more than five years have passed and she has had no recurrence of cancer.

Joan's awareness may have helped to save her life and contribute to her present cured state. Unfortunately, most stories of women with ovarian cancer fit a typical pattern of vague symptoms, delayed treatment, and a poor prognosis. The usual symptoms of ovarian cancer so resemble difficult-to-describe "stomach trouble" that oncologists who treat the disease say the symptoms in most cases of ovarian cancer are drowned in a sea of bicarbonate of soda. Camille's story is typical among women with ovarian cancer.

Camille was in her late fifites when she began to feel as if she had a "puffy stomach." When she saw her internist about this problem she told him, "I'm always bloated and always have a slight case of indigestion." Assuming that she had correctly diagnosed her own problem—stomach trouble—he sent her for a gastrointestinal work-up. All tests were negative and Camille was told she was probably having a nervous reaction to her menopause. "It's age," said the physician. "Your body is changing."

Three months later, Camille felt no better. She had a near-constant stomachache and noticed that her stomach was getting bigger and that antacids had become a steady part of her diet. She went back to her internist, and he sent her to a gynecologist.

The gynecologist whom Camille saw was a specialist in ovarian cancer. It took only a pelvic exam for him to determine that she had a large tumor, and because of her other symptoms, he suspected that the tumor was malignant. During the surgery, his suspicions proved correct. Camille's cancer had spread throughout her ovaries and pelvic region. After surgery, she was started on chemotherapy that has helped her to stay alive and lead a somewhat active life. But her chances for long-term survival are not good.

Ovarian cancer is one of the most dreaded of all the cancers found in the female reproductive system. Only one in every seventy women in the United States, however, will develop ovarian cancer after the age of forty. Surprisingly, there is a rare form of ovarian cancer that is found in young teenagers and even very little girls.

Although ovarian cancer is the fifth leading cause of cancer deaths in women between the ages of thirty-five and forty-five, most women who develop ovarian cancer do so in their mid-fifties. In 1981, about 18,000 women will develop ovarian cancer; for about 11,700 it will be fatal.

The news about ovarian cancer is not all grim. Physicians are investigating new methods, which we discuss later in the chapter, that might assist them in making an earlier diagnosis. Because the problems of early detection have been so great, however, research has focused on treatment. Here there is very good news. Cis-platinum, an effective chemotherapeutic drug, was approved by the Food and Drug Administration in 1979. In cases of ovarian cancer once thought to be untreatable, cis-platinum is a miracle drug. It has done much to prolong the lives of women who develop cancer of the ovaries.

THE OVARIES

The almond-shaped ovaries are small, firm white organs, with a number of spectacular functions. They are responsible for estrogen production, for breast development, for menstruation, and for reproduction. As soon as you enter puberty, the ovaries begin sending out estrogens that change childish figures into the figures of young women. The shape of hips and breasts is largely a function of estrogen.

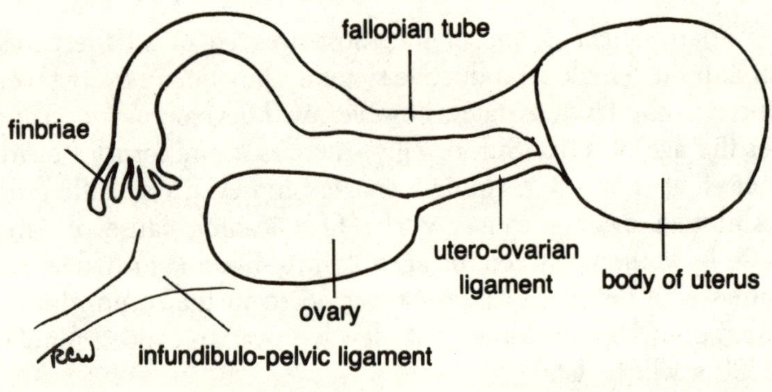

The ovaries. The ovaries, small, almond-shaped organs, are located on either side of the uterus.

When a baby girl is born, her ovaries already contain all the eggs her body will ever need. None of these eggs, however, will leave the ovary before puberty, so none will be available for fertilization before that time. The number of eggs diminishes rapidly in childhood and more slowly as the woman ovulates each month until almost none are left at menopause.

The great director of this masterful production, which takes place in the ovaries, is an intricate network in a region of the brain called the hypothaalmus. It is part of both the nervous system and the hormone system.

During the early days of the menstrual cycle, estrogen levels are low. This low level is a signal for the hypothalamus to "tell" the pituitary to send a follicle-stimulating hormone, FSH, to the ovary. Once FSH goes to the ovary, the cells of the follicle begin producing estrogen. The follicle is an egg-carrying case. There are many follicles in the ovary, but only one seems to get called up to the surface. Just how or why that one is selected is not known. It carries the egg that can one day be fertilized. The time it takes for a developing follicle to move the egg to the surface of the ovary is about fourteen days. (See the illustration.)

During the middle of your ovulation cycle, which would be about day 14 after the first day of your menstrual cycle, the egg-carrying follicle ruptures and releases the egg inside, and the egg now moves down the fallopian tube. This rupture also releases a small amount of blood, which may irritate the (inner) lining of the abdomen. You might even feel a sharp pain. If you are one of those women aware of this pain, then you know instinctively that you are ovulating. This phenomenon is called *mittelschmerz,* the German word for middle pain.

After the follicle ruptures, the egg will head for the fallopian tube; then either of two events might take place: If the egg meets the sperm and is fertilized, in less than a week it will move down into the uterus and there grow into a developing embryo. If conception does not take place, the egg will be shed in menstruation.

While the egg is traveling, the ruptured follicle cyst is undergoing a change. Once a producer of estrogen—while it carried its egg—it now takes on a new function. As if to protect the egg it has given up, it prepares the uterus for an anticipated pregnancy. How does this happen?

Estrogen levels are high around ovulation. These high levels are a sign to the hypothalamus that they must be balanced with another hormone, progesterone. The hypothalamus signals the pituitary, which sends LH, luteinizing hormone, to the follicle. With LH, the follicles turns into what is called a corpus luteum. One of the reasons it is called a corpus luteum after the productin of LH has to do with its color: As it gets older the follicle turns yellow, and corpus luteum means "yellow body." The yellow color comes from beta carotene—vitamin A—also found in yellow and yellow-green vegetables.

The follicle is now devoid of its very minute egg, yet it continues to function in the reproductive cycle. It produces progesterone as well as estrogen, and the combination of these hormones prepares the uterine lining to house a growing embryo and fetus. The uterine lining thickens as it waits for a sperm and egg—united in conception—to arrive.

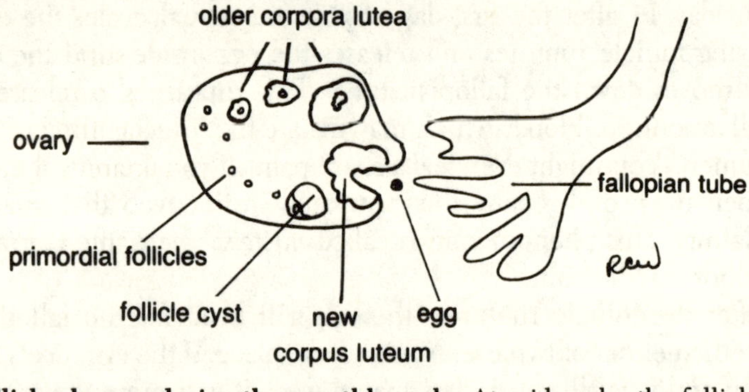

Follicle changes during the monthly cycle. At mid-cycle, the follicle cyst ruptures and releases the egg, which moves down the fallopian tube.

If conception takes place, the corpus luteum plays a vital role in the first few weeks of pregnancy by giving hormonal support to the growing fetus.

Of course, if the tiny egg released by the follicle cyst does not meet with a sperm, conception does not take place. The build-up of cells in the uterine lining is shed in menstruation about two weeks after midcycle. Menstruation has been called "the tears of a frustrated uterus."

During menstruation, the corpus luteum diminishes in size, and after some length of time—it may be several months—the yellow color fades and the corpus luteum turns into the whitish corpus albicans (the Latin *albus* means "white"). Estrogen and progesterone levels are declining at menstruation. It is now up to the brain to send out releasing factors to begin the cycle of estrogen production again.

Estrogen is produced primarily by the ovaries. It has multiple complex functions until its effects are withdrawn during the time of menopause. It is at this time, when estrogen production practically ceases, that the ovaries harbor the hidden hazard of cancer. Just why this is true, however, is not known. Why is it that some women get ovarian cancer and others do not? It has been very difficult to pinpoint just what type of woman is at risk for developing ovarian cancer. Thus far, it has been suggested that women whose mothers, sisters, or close relatives had ovarian cancer are at somewhat greater risk for developing the disease. Some studies have shown that other women at risk are those who are infertile or who have endometriosis.

An Egyptian researcher has suggested that incessant ovulation, without intervening pregnancy to block ovulation for nine or more months at a stretch, may lead to some change in the surface of the ovary that predisposes one to ovarian cancer. Although his argument is tenuous, statistical data about comparative reproductive activity in various worldwide groups of women tend to support this view.

Since ovarian cancer is found primarily in industrialized societies, some epidemiological research studies have suggested that it might be related to an environmental factor. Yet, in highly industrialized Japan, ovarian cancer rates are among the lowest in the world.

One's chances of ovarian cancer increase with age, as the chart indicates.

CHANCE OF CONTRACTING OVARIAN CANCER

Age	
Under 12	Because there are rare forms of ovarian cancer that young girls develop, an ovarian enlargement is frequently malignant.
12–30	Most ovarian enlargements are functional cysts (follicle or corpus luteum) that regress.
35–50	Chances for ovarian cancer rise considerably.
Over 50	There is nearly a 50 percent chance that an ovarian enlargement is malignant.

SYMPTOMS OF OVARIAN CANCER

When you cannot adequately determine if you are at risk for a disease, you should make all the more certain that you are at least aware of the symptoms. With ovarian cancer, as mentioned before, the symptoms are so insidious that detection has been difficult. You should report any ongoing symptoms of stomach trouble, even vague ones, to your physician immediately.

As in Camille's story, the ovarian cancer often produces a bloated feeling in the stomach. This is partly due to fluid accumulating in the abdominal cavity. Fluid accumulates because the tumor produces it. You might even notice that your stomach is becoming puffy; this is because the tumor is beginning to swell.

You might have a gassy feeling and find yourself belching. You will feel nauseated occasionally. There is enough space around the ovary so that it can become quite large before it actually impinges on other organs and causes true pain.

Because these symptoms all seem to relate to stomach problems rather than pelvic problems, most women go first to an internist for treatment. It is while the internist conducts gastrointestinal investigations, only to find nothing, that precious time is lost. Frequently six months will pass before a woman with ovarian cancer sees a gynecologist who correctly diagnoses the problem.

DETECTING OVARIAN CANCER

A tumor mass on an ovary can be felt and a physician usually can detect it during a regular exam, but only in the later stages. In the early stages a tumor mass on the ovary may be felt, but if you have vague stomach problems and see an internist as opposed to a gynecologist, you should still *insist* upon a pelvic exam. If there is a tumor present, it might be large enough for your physician to feel it. The tumor often extends behind the uterus and in front of the rectum, filling a space called the *cul-de-sac*.

In most cases if a surgeon suspects ovarian cancer you will be hospitalized, and laparotomy, which is the technical term for exploratory surgery, will be scheduled. Laparotomy usually involves a five-inch incision below the navel. Definite diagnosis can only be made at the time of surgery, so you will be scheduled for surgery with the understanding that if cancer is found, the physician will take the necessary steps to remove all diseased organs.

There may be cases in which physicians can determine whether a tumor is benign or malignant through other techniques. These other techniques include ultrasound, paracentesis, and laparoscopy.

Ultrasound, also called sonography or "sonar," is based on echos. With ultrasound, you will be asked to drink a number of glasses of water throughout the day and refrain from emptying your bladder. With the fluid accumulation in the bladder, you will then have a sonogram made. During the test, you lie still on a table, and a transducer, a microphone-like device, is placed on your stomach. The transducer produces a sound wave that bounces off the tumor site and is recorded on a TV screen. The principle is the same as in sonar for detecting submarines. Ultrasound can tell a physician not just the size of a tumor and its location, but also its consistency. A solid malignant tumor has a different consistency from a benign cyst. Even after ultrasound, however, it may still be advisable to have exploratory surgery. The primary advantage of sonar for you is in at least knowing the likelihood of the tumor's being benign or malignant before the surgery.

Paracentesis is another technique that is sometimes useful in an initial diagnosis. It is usually performed by an internist and can be done in his or her office. In this procedure, a hollow needle is inserted into the abdomen and fluid is withdrawn. By analyzing the fluid, it can sometimes be determined whether or not malignant cells exist. Since this procedure delays definitive diagnosis, some physicians encourage immediate surgery.

Laparoscopy is a minor surgical procedure. It involves making an incision in the navel into which a special ultraslim telescope is inserted. A gynecologist usually uses this procedure to rule out the possibility of a malignancy. Through the telescope, he or she can actually see the ovaries and tell whether or not they are normal in size and shape. This is especially useful for testing a younger woman who has an enlarged ovary. With this technique, a gynecologist often can tell whether or not you have a small fibroid tumor or an ovarian enlargement. Laparoscopy is rarely used when ovarian cancer is suspected, however, since full visualizational exploratory surgery will be necessary for the latter.

If you or your internist suspect ovarian cancer, it is important that you find a surgeon trained in gynecological oncology. Many obstetricians and gynecologists routinely refer women to specialists in this field because ovarian cancer can be so difficult to treat. Unlike most other forms of cancer, ovarian tumors are in a class by themselves. There is no such thing as a standard ovarian tumor; there are at least thirty different varieties of tumors, some which are fatal within several months. A trained gynecologic oncologist is familiar with the different tumor varieties and often is able to provide treatments that are not usually available at smaller hospitals. The story of Harumi is a case in point.

Harumi was a laboratory technician who had come to America from Japan. She was the type of worker whose speed and proficiency amazed her coworkers. When she began having vague stomach pains, she ignored the symptoms and continued her work. When she felt too sick to continue with her job, she saw an internist. He told her that she had either an ectopic pregnancy (in which the fetus is growing outside its proper place in the uterus) or endometriosis. Harumi was sent to a gynecologist who admitted her for surgery at a small suburban hospital.

At the time of surgery, the surgeon found a tumor so large and so extensive that he merely took a portion of it, gave it to a pathologist, and closed the incision without attempting to remove it. The pathologist at the hospital diagnosed Harumi as having a rare and usually fatal form of ovarian canner. Harumi's husband was told that there was virtually nothing that could be done to save his wife, but that she would be kept comfortable and given heavy doses of morphine until she died.

A research scientist himself, Harumi's husband would not accept the pathologist's diagnosis and had his wife transferred immediately to a teaching hospital in New York City. At that hospital, Harumi's tumor was again analyzed by a pathologist. Harumi did have ovarian cancer, but it was not the rare tumor that she had been told would be fatal within a matter of months. Harumi was started on treatment with an experimental chemotherapeutic drug that shrank the tumor. In three months she was again operated on, and the surgeon was able to remove the remaining part of the tumor. Although she needed intense treatment for six months, Harumi was then able to go back to her normal life. She could enjoy her family, her friends, and her work. Harumi lived two years beyond the expectations of the physicians who originally treated her.

TREATING OVARIAN CANCER

The progress of cancer is often considered in stages, and in early stages treatment is frequently less extensive than in later ones. With ovarian cancer, the disease is almost never spotted in the earliest stage, which physicians call Stage I. A source chart on cancer patients' survival made by the American Cancer Society, *Cancer Statistics, 1981* noted that between 1970 and 1973, only 25 percent of the cases of ovarian cancer were diagnosed during this initial stage, 6 percent at the regionalized stage, and 64 percent in distant metastases. Despite these figures, physicians who normally treat ovarian cancer say that less than 10 percent of women are diagnosed in an early enough stage for long-term survival. It is believed by physicians that a full 90 percent diagnosed already have distant metastases. Why the discrepancies? American Cancer Society statistics are based on various reporting methods and hospital charts. Physicians who regularly treat ovarian cancer feel that it is not uncommon for a benign ovarian tumor to be misdiagnosed, especially in smaller hospitals that see fewer of these tumors. With this margin of error, the statistics vary.

Stage I means that cancer is detected only in the ovaries and has not yet spread to other organs. Stage II means that the cancer has spread to the pelvic tissues and/or the uterus and fallopian tubes. In Stage III it has spread to regions outside the pelvis, such as the upper abdomen, and in Stage IV it has spread to distant parts of the body such as the chest.

Treatment, whether at Stage I or Stage IV, usually is surgery combined with chemotherapy. Surgery for ovarian cancer generally will include removal of both ovaries and/or fallopian tubes, all or part of the uterus (the cancer cells frequently travel to that area), and the omentum, a fatty tissue in the upper abdomen that is adjacent to the large intestine and often the site for metastases.

Even if the cancer appears to be confined to just one ovary, surgeons familiar with the disease feel it is best to remove the uterus and both ovaries and fallopian tubes. At the time of surgery, if the surgeon sees any tumor deposits or can feel them in other areas, they too will be removed.

Chemotherapy for ovarian cancer involves the use of a new drug, cis-platinum (DDP, cis dichlorodiammine platinum). The drug has proved to be so effective when used in combination with other drugs such as adriamycin, cytoxan, thio-tepa, and hexamethylmeamine that there is a response rate of close to 70 percent in tumors that once were thought to be untreatable. This means that almost 70 percent of the tumors have responded to the drug with some obvious reduction in tumor size. Because the crucial problem of early diagnosis is still unsolved, finding a drug like cis-platinum that improves the response rate for such a serious disease is a major step forward.

Other drugs used to treat ovarian cancer include alkylating agents such as cytoxan, melphalan, and thio-tepa. These are less toxic and easier to tolerate than cis-platinum and adriamycin, but also less effective when used alone. All the drugs used for treatment of ovarian cancer, however, are harsh on the system and difficult to tolerate. You will experience severe nausea and vomiting, and most antinausea drugs will not help. Marijuana and some of its synthetic analogues appear to reduce these unpleasant side effects—some women have said "by a bit"; others say "tremendously." (For more about the side effects of chemotherapy, see Chapter 11.)

If you have ovarian cancer, find a hospital that either is a major cancer center or has physicians who have had experience using newer drugs. You may feel like a guinea pig—and resent it—while using a drug in its experimental stages, but keep in mind that during the investigative period in developing new drugs, there is very close surveillance of both patient and investigator. You and your physician are checked not only by the federal government, but by the special staff at the teaching hospitals where these drugs are used. If there is a promising new drug, you might well consider going to a hospital that has access to it. We are not suggesting you give every new drug a try. Each situation must be evaluated separately. With ovarian cancer, however, since the disease generally is so far along when it is found, gambling on a new drug might mean the difference between life and death.

Some women feel that they would rather wait until a drug is approved and then have a doctor at their local hospital administer it. The fact is that a physician who has not been using the drug regularly can do you more harm than good. Cis-platinum has extremely harsh side effects and can damage the kidneys and other organs. You owe it to yourself to have it administered by professionals who know how to use it and how to regulate and monitor the dosages. Physicians in hospitals in suburban communities rarely have enough patients with a particular type of ovarian cancer to have gained the experience needed to learn about the drug and its side effects.

Radiation treatment, once a common follow-up to surgery, is rarely used today for treating ovarian cancer. Chemotherapy has proved so effective that radiation therapy in most cases should be considered obsolete. Some physicians, however, accustomed to using radiation as a traditional treatment method, have resisted chemotherapy, and sometimes a woman will request radiation because she is afraid of chemotherapy. A physician might consent to her wishes by rationalizing that it is better than nothing. In fact, radiation therapy might be *worse* than nothing. Radiation therapy often damages the bone marrow reserves that a woman might need later on to make blood cells if she eventually does undergo chemotherapy. Today chemotherapy becomes crucial when the disease spreads. It is not unusual to be given surgery and then need chemotherapy for three or four years.

Treatment for ovarian cancer is unpleasant. It is perhaps the most difficult of all types of female cancers to adjust to, both physically and emotionally. Because it has such a poor prognosis, and because its symptoms make it so difficult to detect, we urge you again to be aware of the symptoms and to make certain that you receive a thorough check-up if you have any doubt whatever about the possibility of having this disease.

Questioning a physician about your health is an indication that you are concerned and aware and want to be informed. It is important for you to let a physician know that you want to participate in your own health-care decisions. If you are seeing a gynecologic oncologist because you or your physician suspects you have ovarian cancer, you might consider asking the following questions: How often do you treat ovarian cancer? (The answer should be at least one new case each month if the physician is at a teaching hospital.) What chemotherapeutic drugs do you use for follow-up treatment? (See chart on page 194.) How long has your oncology team had access to them? (In most teaching hospitals this should not be a concern.)

CANCER OF THE FALLOPIAN TUBES

This is the rarest of all cancers found in female reproductive organs—so rare that no one knows its cause or whether a particular group is at risk. It usually is diagnosed only in older women during a pelvic exam in which the physician will feel a tubal enlargement. In exceptional instances, cells shed from the tumor might pass through the uterus and be detected by a cytologist in a Pap smear taken from the cervix.

Treatment for fallopian cancer is similar to treatment of ovarian cancer: surgery and chemotherapy. In most cases the prognosis is poor, but as treatment of ovarian cancer improves, women with fallopian-tube cancer will benefit as well.

NON-MALIGNANT OVARIAN CONDITIONS

If you are seeing any physician or a gynecologic oncologist for a routine check-up, ask whether he or she felt anything unusual in your ovaries or uterus. Fibroids and cysts are common, but you should be informed if you have them.

Fibroids are not related to ovarian cancer in any way. They often differ in consistency from ovarian tumors and generally grow from muscle and connective tissue. They are solid, whereas ovarian tumors are often cystic, that is, fluidlike in consistency. Some ovarian tumors are solid, and it is very difficult to tell them apart from fibroids except by exploratory surgery, but they are rare. Usually through making a pelvic exam, using sonar, and watching your condition your physician can distinguish a fibroid from an ovarian tumor. After a WNET television special, "The Story of Joan Robinson," many women became concerned about the possibility of misdiagnosis. (Mrs. Robinson was told she had a fibroid when actually she had ovarian cancer.) The story of Juliette is typical.

Juliette had been having bladder problems. She saw her gynecologist, who sent her to a urologist. The urologist told her the

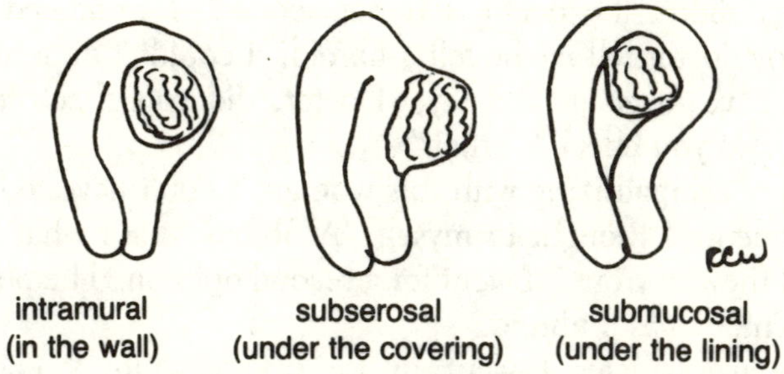

Fibroids. Fibroids are benign growths that generally grow from muscle or connective tissue. They are not related to ovarian cancer in any way. The illustration above shows the three usual locations of the fibroids within the uterus.

problem was caused by a large fibroid pushing up against her bladder. She returned to the gynecologist, who told her he had suspected all along that she had a slow growing fibroid but only wanted confirmation from the urologist. Juliette was quite upset that the gynecologist had never told *her* that she had a fibroid. When she mentioned this to the physician, he said, "I didn't want to worry you. I've been watching it for several years now. It should be removed, but I am certain it is nothing more than a fibroid."

Soon afterward, Juliette saw the documentary television program about Joan Robinson. "It was the first television program I had ever seen about cancer. You can imagine what I felt like when, right in the beginning of the show, I heard this woman—now dead—say that her doctor told her she had nothing more than a rapidly growing fibroid and it turned out to be ovarian cancer. When she asked him how he knew about it, he just told her, 'Because I felt it on your last visit.'

"'Why didn't the doctor tell her sooner?' I wondered. 'Why didn't my doctor tell *me* he felt a fibroid?' I couldn't understand it. Do we have to go in and say, 'Doctor, did you check for this? Doctor, did you check for that?'

"As I'm sympathizing with this woman, I don't have to tell you that suddenly I thought to myself, 'A fibroid, that's what I have. What if they're wrong?' I went for a second opinion. The physician assured me it was a fibroid.

"Two weeks later I went in for my operation," continued Juliette. "Despite the reassurances, despite the second opinion, until I was out of the operating room and they told me, 'You are fine,' I didn't have a peaceful night's sleep."

Ovarian Cysts

The ovaries regularly produce fluid-filled sacs of different sizes, the most common of which is the follicle cyst. These normally grow and regress during the ovulation and menstrual cycles. Sometimes a follicle cyst will not regress and can become relatively large, the size of a lemon. Although it is also possible for a cyst of the corpus luteum to persist, this happens much less often—usually only during a pregnancy.

If a physician feels a cyst during a pelvic exam, he or she will assume that with the close of the menstrual cycle, the cyst will regress. No one knows for certain, however, why it is that some cysts do not regress. Sometimes the persistent cyst will cause you to feel dizzy and nauseated. Sometimes the cyst will twist or rupture, causing pain.

A cyst that does not regress naturally after two menstrual cycles probably needs to be surgically removed. In the past some physicians have used hormonal therapy for ovarian cysts. Never consent to this treatment. There is no logical basis for this treatment and it has been proven worthless.

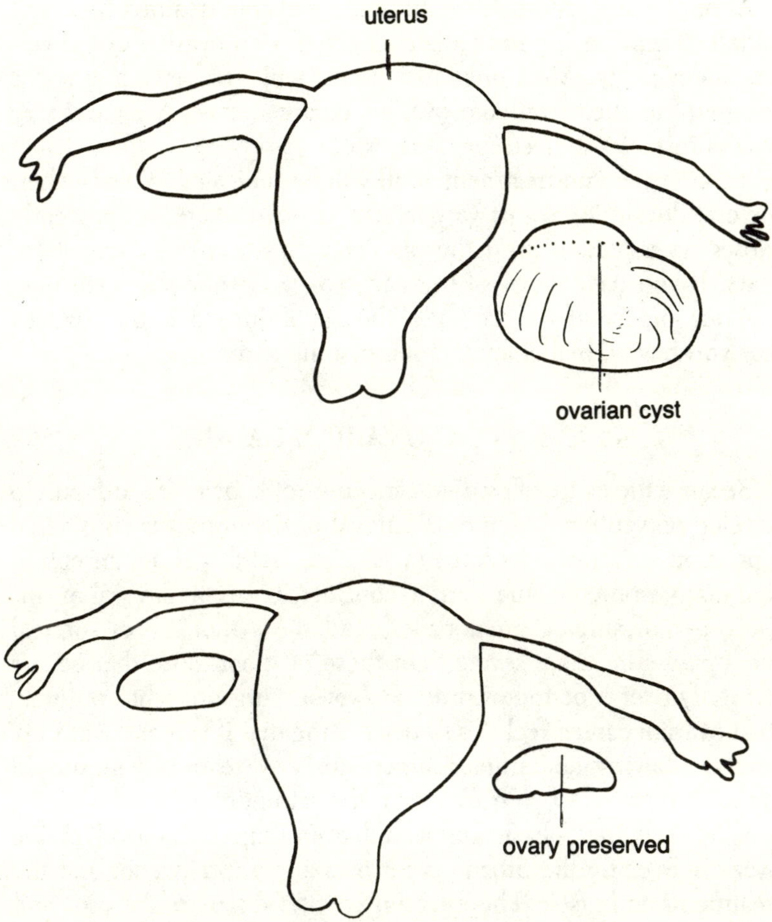

Removal of an ovarian cyst. The ovaries regularly produce fluid-filled sacs, called cysts, which grow and regress during the course of the menstrual cycle. If they do not regress, surgery may sometimes (though not always) be necessary. The illustrations show that a cyst may be removed without removing the ovary.

Although surgery might be the most sensible treatment, do not be talked into having immediate surgery for an ovarian cyst if you are under thirty. Most physicians today will first perform a sonar test that can help evaluate ovarian enlargements. A laparoscopy may eliminate the need for more extensive surgery.

In rare cases, no treatment at all will be indicated. This is when the cyst does not grow or vary in size; it is just there, it apparently causes no problems, and the physician has been watching it for years. If you have a cyst of this sort, you and your physician may rule out surgery. If you are under the age of thirty-five, the chances that you have a malignant ovarian cyst are slim.

PREVENTING OVARIAN CANCER

Because the cause of ovarian cancer is not known, it is difficult to develop preventive measures. Removal of the ovaries is considered a preventive measure by some physicians, but this is not an option that many women would want to consider. Ovarian removal means the onset of surgical menopause, and the symptoms of surgical menopause are more severe than those of menopause that occurs naturally over a period of time. However, surgeons who routinely treat ovarian cancer feel it is so devastating that if you are over forty and are having abdominal surgery for any reason, you should consider removal of your ovaries at the same time.

Why is it that physicians would even suggest removal of the ovaries? Because the prognosis for ovarian cancer is poor and the treatments so harsh. (The estrogen chapter discusses the pros and cons of ovarian removal.) If you are high risk and decide against ovarian removal, be aware of any unusual stomach trouble. Find a skilled gynecologic oncologist who has access to sonar equipment. Go for routine check-ups. Be aware!

Chapter Eight

Estrogen, Menopause, and Cancer

Sondra had heard all the horror stories about menopause from her mother. Because she associated menopause with hot flashes, depression, and old wrinkled skin, she made up her mind that she would not suffer through this ordeal. By age forty, she had convinced herself that when menopause approached, she would be first on the estrogen-pill line. That was five years ago. Now Sondra is in menopause. After reading about some of the serious side effects of estrogen, she has had second thoughts about the drug. In fact, Sondra became so involved with the question of estrogen-replacement therapy that, she said, "before I even realized it, I was in menopause, living through it, without all the so-called side effects."

Serena, on the other hand, did have serious menopausal symptoms. She had such severe night sweats that she admitted to waking up in what she described as "a pool of water." Nonetheless, Serena also rejected estrogens.

Camille was worried about the relationship of estrogen to cancer, but she felt an absolute need for estrogen pills. Camille found a physician who prescribed the pills but watched her very carefully. She took the precautions suggested by her physician and the drug manufacturers (all estrogen pills today are labeled with precautions). Now, after two years on estrogen, she is beginning to cut down on the drug. Within a few months, she may stop taking it altogether. She feels, however, that it helped her through menopause.

Estrogen-replacement therapy is one of the most controversial issues facing women today. For years physicians believed that they could prevent menopausal miseries by replacing the natural hormone estrogen, which a woman's ovaries almost completely stop producing during menopause, with supplemental estrogen.

According to a *New York Times* report, prior to 1975, when the studies linking estrogen to endometrial cancer were first publicized, about twenty million prescriptions for the drug were filled annually. Today more than thirty million American women are past menopause with fewer than seven million using estrogen supplements. Why?

In addition to the studies linking exogenous estrogens—that is, hormone pills or injections—to cancer, there has been a total reevaluation of the effectiveness of estrogen in the treatment of menopausal symptoms. Women and physicians are now taking a much closer look at what for years was an accepted practice.

ESTROGEN AND MENOPAUSE

The hormone estrogen is produced naturally within a woman's body in a number of ways. The adrenal gland furnishes a small amount, and some also is made from cholesterol in a process called peripheral conversion in fat and other substances. Most estrogen, however, comes from the ovaries, where it is produced each month by the follicle after it has ruptured.

Estrogen is the prototypical female hormone. When a young girl begins to produce it at puberty, it stimulates the development of her body, giving shape to her hips and breasts, regulating bone growth, and promoting secretions that keep her vagina moist. It also is one of the keys to reproduction. Each month, the estrogen helps prepare the lining of the uterus, the endometrium, to receive the egg from the follicle should it be fertilized. If the egg is not fertilized, then the prepared lining will be shed, producing the bloody discharge called menstruation (from *mensis*, the Latin word for "month"). From the time a woman begins to have regular periods, her whole body is in tune with her monthly cycle of estrogen production. (See Chapter 7 on the ovaries for a detailed discussion of the estrogen cycle.)

At about age forty-five or fifty, a woman's ovaries begin to shrink, and production of estrogen from the ovaries, the body's major source of the hormone, gradually ceases. In turn, the uterus stops receiving the hormonal signals to prepare itself for a fertilized egg, and the monthly periods come to an end. This profound change of life is called menopause (from the Greek *men*, or "month," and *pauein*, "to cause to cease"). Because the process takes place over a period of time, perhaps several years, it is possible for a woman to conceive at this time. "Change of life babies" are not unknown.

Menopause is a perfectly natural female function, but one that has a number of unhappy side effects. They are described, almost invariably, as hot flashes, vaginal dryness, wrinkled skin, irritability, and depression—the last of which may actually be related to other factors. Because menopause occurs gradually, some women naturally adjust to the decrease in estrogen in their bodies without experiencing any side effects. For those who do not adjust easily, however, estrogen-replacement therapy was used.

Menopause does not always occur naturally. Surgical menopause occurs when a woman has her ovaries removed. Surgical menopause is an abrupt shock to the system, and the use of estrogen replacement in this instance may well be advisable and necessary.

Both synthetic and natural hormones have been used in estrogen replacement therapy. Synthetic estrogens are chemical substances that have effects similar to those of natural estrogens. For example, diethylstilbesterol (DES) has a different molecular shape from estrogen, but parts of the body cannot tell the two substances apart, so the synthetic hormone produces the same effects as the natural one. Other substances, derived from animals, are either identical or almost identical to the estrogen produced by human ovaries, and so they are termed "natural estrogens." There are also some "semisynthetic" estrogens, which are derived from hormonal or steroid molecules that have been gathered from animal or even plant sources, such as the Mexican sweet potato. Many of the hormones in birth control pills are derived from these.

ESTROGEN-REPLACEMENT THEORY AND MENOPAUSAL SIDE EFFECTS

Women's reasons for wanting estrogen-replacement therapy (ERT) generally fall into two categories, emotional and physical. From the emotional point of view, it was believed—and still is by many physicians—that estrogen can relieve the symptoms of depression in menopause. But does menopause really cause depression? Recent studies indicate that menopausal depression is a myth.

In her book *Unfinished Business,* Maggie Scarf reports on women who were treated with estrogen for years because of depression. In Chapter Fifteen, telling the story of Doris Nordlund, Mrs. Scarf quotes Doris as saying, "The doctors told me that menopause was what the whole thing was all about. They kept saying, 'Here, take a few drops of femininity and then you can just run along.' And so, of course, that's what I did. But I just kept getting sicker and sicker."

For Doris Nordlund, estrogenic substances of all sorts had been supplied; they were her medicine, says Mrs. Scarf. It was never suggested to her—not, at least, until she nearly died of it—that her disease pertained less to her ovaries and her reproductive system than to her entire life, her entire way of being. Mrs. Scarf interviewed Mrs. Nordlund while she was a patient at Yale University's School of Medicine, the Dana Psychiatric Institute, where she was brought after an almost lethal suicide try.

"Women expect menopausal symptoms because their doctors tell them they will have them," Mrs. Scarf writes. "Yet for those who do experience a depression, it isn't because of menopause, it is because of things in their own lives that they are not happy about. Women say it's about hormones, but it isn't," she declares.

Mrs. Scarf's conclusions are supported by other investigations. Several of these studies were cited in a 1979 article in the *Journal of the American Medical Association*, "The Myth of Involutional Melancholiea" by Dr. Myrna Weissman of the Yale Research Depression Unit. For example, a community survey in England of more than 600 women of premenopausal and menopausal ages concluded that "there is no direct relationship between depression and menopausal states." In another study of 800 women between the ages of thirty-eight and sixty, conducted from 1968 to 1970, the findings were the same: No significant differences that could be attributed to menopause were observed in the rates of mental illness or depression for women of different ages.

Dr. Weissman herself conducted a similar study of women in New Haven from 1967 to 1976. In interviews and reinterviews, the same results were found. If anything, the evidence pointed the other way: The rates of depressive symptoms were highest among women *younger* than thirty-five, and they tended to decrease gradually with age. This study concludes that "research findings do not support an increased prevalence of depression around the menopausal years." A special panel on estrogen use of the National Institutes of Health also concluded in 1979 that there was no association between menopause and depression.

Thus if you feel that you need estrogen for a physical reason, you might consider it. But for severe depression, there just is not sufficient evidence that menopause actually causes it or that estrogen can relieve it.

Can estrogen-replacement therapy relieve the physical symptoms associated with menopause—vaginal dryness, hot flashes, thinning of the bones, and wrinkled skin? Yes, it does relieve some of these, and physicians believe it is more effective than other remedies.

The benefits of estrogen therapy, however, should be weighed against the accumulating evidence that it promotes cancer, and the fact that other remedies *can* help. For example, vaginal dryness can make sexual intercourse painful, but women can use a safe, simple, water-soluble lubricant or a vaginal cream without estrogen in it. Vaginal creams containing estrogen can be as effective as estrogens that are taken orally, but because the creams are absorbed by the body they may be harmful. As for wrinkles in the skin, estrogen creams may puff out the little lines under the eyes a bit, but it is unlikely that any long-lasting benefit will be gained. Face creams with estrogen may not be as potentially harmful as vaginal creams that are absorbed internally; still, most of these have been withdrawn from the market.

Estrogen-replacement therapy has another dependable, positive effect, reducing the dangers posed to older women by progressive osteoporosis (bone thinning). Women with osteoporosis become shorter and shorter as their spine and long bones give less and less support, and they are much more likely than most people to suffer fractures in comparatively minor accidents. Fractured hips are especially dangerous. Hip fractures have so many complications that there is a 15 percent chance of death within three months; that is, one woman in seven will die within ninety days. Estrogen therapy, if started within a few years of menopause, blocks the loss of bone from osteoporosis and despite some natural vitamin cures only estrogen is known to prevent bone loss.

A study of 567 women, reported in *The New England Journal of Medicine* in 1980, showed that estrogen therapy lowered the risk of fractures to the hip and lower arm by 50 to 60 percent among women who had been taking estrogen supplements for six years or more. In this area, then, estrogen definitely reduces the dangers of a life-threatening condition. But consider the tradeoff.

Finally, it has been suggested that estrogen therapy might help prevent heart attacks. This suggestion was based on the observation that heart attacks from coronary artery disease are much less frequent among white women before menopause than among white men of similar age, and that the incidence of heart attacks among women increased following menopause. Some physicians felt the differences in estrogen levels explained this pattern and that use of estrogen supplements might help delay or prevent hardening of the arteries. All this is speculative, however; there is, as yet, no proof that estrogen pills can prevent heart attacks. Estrogen does, however, change the levels of fatty substances in the blood and thus protects the small blood vessels of the heart. (Some researchers suggest the same effect from drinking two glasses of wine a day.)

ESTROGEN AND CANCER

The link between estrogen and cancer has been a matter of some controversy in medical circles. On November 16, 1978, *The New England Journal of Medicine* reported a study conducted by Drs. Ralph Horwitz and Alvan Feinstein at the Yale University School of Medicine which concluded that "The magnitude of association between estrogens and endometrial cancer has been greatly overestimated because of detection bias. . . ." By January 4, 1979 the same journal reported on a large case control study by Dr. Carlos M. F. Atunes *et al.* that found "The overall risk of endometrial carcinoma was sixfold for estrogen users as compared with nonusers . . ." They noted that "the clinical implications of this study directly concern the use of estrogen replacement therapy. "Despite the debate within medical circles, there are strong associations between estrogen and endometrial cancer.

Some studies seem to confirm the risk of cancer, which apparently is greatest three years and later after a woman has begun to take synthetic or natural estrogens by mouth or injection. The increased cancer risk was noted by the National Institute of Health panel on estrogen. Even the manufacturer who packages estrogen includes a statement about the risk of cancer to women taking estrogen. The longer you take estrogen, the greater the risk.

If you do not take estrogen supplements, your chances of developing endometrial cancer are about one in 1,000; if you do take estrogen, your chances may increase threefold after several years.

The malignant precursor, endometrial hyperplasia, should also be kept in mind when considering ERT. In some 15 to 20 percent of the women who have endometrial hyperplasia, an endometrial cancer eventually will develop. In most cases of endometrial hyperplasia, the condition arises without the use of estrogen supplements and may reflect a natural tendency of the lining of the uterus to produce this condition or a response to estrogen being produced in the body. When endometrial hyperplasia is found in this way, in a woman who no longer wants or is able to bear children, the usual treatment is hysterectomy because of the known risk of developing endometrial cancer.

However, natural or synthetic estrogens taken by mouth or injection will induce endometrial hyperplasia in some women. Whether they are at the same risk for developing a subsequent cancer of the endometrium as those in whom hyperplasia arises without exogenous estrogens is not conclusively known at this time.

Many people also fear that estrogen-replacement therapy may increase the risk of breast cancer, but again the data are not dependable. In the United States two studies, each carefully conducted, came to opposite conclusions. One indicated a slight increase in breast cancer among women taking estrogen; the other found no relationship between estrogen therapy and incidence of breast cancer. At an international conference in 1980 on breast cancer, however, the consensus was that estrogen does play a role in cases of the disease. Quoting the Special Report on the Epidemiology and Etiology of Breast Cancer from the meeting of the Multi-Disciplinary Project on Breast Cancer of the International Union Against Cancer, held at Leeds Castle, England, in June 1980, *The New England Journal of Medicine* stated, "There is evidence that after a ten- to fifteen-year latency period, there is an increased risk of breast cancer in women who have used non-contraceptive estrogens at the time of menopause. Use for more than two to five years does not seem to be required for enhanced risk to occur, indicating a relationship between estrogen and breast cancer in that some breast cancers—predominantly in younger women who have not reached menopause—are treated by removal of the ovaries. Thus deprived of most of their estrogen supplies, these patients do better." Drugs that block the effects of estrogen also are used in some breast cancer cases. Neither of these treatments, however, proves that estrogen actually causes breast cancer, though they do imply that at least some breast cancers have "estrogen receptors"—cellular mechanisms that respond to estrogen.

Some leading medical authorities have advocated that when estrogen-replacement therapy is used, still another hormone be added to lessen the risk of endometrial cancer. They believe that progesterone, the ovarian hormone of the second part of the normal menstrual cycle, or a progestagen (a progesterone-like substance) can be given to women taking estrogen replacement and substantially reduce or eliminate the risk of endometrial cancer. When this plan is followed, the estrogen pill is given daily for most of the month and the progestagen pill for about one week. An added nuisance is occasional bleeding like a menstrual period. But at the time of this writing there have been no endometrial cancers reported in women treated this way. Another safeguard is periodic biopsies of the uterus, looking for endometrial cancer precursors.

Would the use of a progestagen expose you to some other hazard or cancer unknown at this time? Maybe. The answer isn't known yet. On the plus side: No cancer related to progestagens has been described, and progestagens are used in the *treatment* of endometrial and some other cancers. No one knows, however, what the long-term effects of progestagens might be. Would it be better to stay clear of them until more is known? This question takes us back to the severity and quality of a woman's menopausal symptoms, to the woman herself and her needs, and to the physician and his or her opinions.

DECIDING WHAT TO DO

The theory behind this book is that *all* medical decisions should be made by a woman *in cooperation with* her physician. Some risks may be worth taking and others may not, and what is worthwhile for one person may not be worthwhile for another. Each woman will have to decide what is right for her, after consulting with her physician and considering all the factors in her particular situation.

We cannot stress enough how important it is for a woman to learn to say "*No*" when she does not feel comfortable with a particular drug. Conversely, if you and your physician decide that you really need estrogens (or any other treatment, for that matter), do not be intimidated by friends or media reports opposed to estrogen use. Just be certain that you are fully informed about the potential risks and benefits of estrogen therapy.

You should read the warnings that the Food and Drug Administration has required manufacturers to include with prescriptions for estrogen pills. Some pharmacists say that many women will take the pills and say, "No, thank you" to the manufacturer's insert. But any woman using estrogen owes it to herself to read this notice. It lists the dangers of estrogen, including the risks of cancer of the endometrium, vagina, breast, and liver, as well as gallbladder disease and abnormal blood clotting. It also lists side effects such as nausea and vomiting, vaginal bleeding, and other effects on the breasts and uterus. All these should be discussed in advance with your physician.

Anyone who is taking estrogen also should be aware that in a recommendation to physicians in 1976, the Food and Drug Administration suggested that women should receive the lowest possible dosage, perhaps 0.3 to 0.625 milligrams a day. It should be stressed that all women on ERT have endometrial biopsies at least once a year!

And finally, when considering the pros and cons of estrogen-replacement therapy, you should remember that the National Institute of Health, during its estrogen panel studies in 1979, concluded that the woman herself should be the ultimate judge in deciding whether or not to take estrogen supplements. How do you decide? Weigh the risks and the benefits in your own case—and make certain your thinking is not clouded by myths.

RECOMMENDED ARTICLES

Mann JI. Progestogens in cardiovascular diseases: an introduction to the epidemiologic data. *American Journal of Obstetrics and Gynecology* 142:752–7.

Meade TW. Effects of progestogens on the cardiovascular system. *American Journal of Obstetrics and Gynecology* 142:776–80.

Chapter Nine

The Vulva and the Vagina

Moo loved children. She had six of her own and cared for five nieces and nephews in her large San Francisco home. Moo also loved to travel and often accompanied her husband on his business trips. When she developed a mild but constant itch around her vagina, she tried every possible home remedy. Finally it began to interfere with her sex life, so she went to a gynecologist.

The gynecologist saw immediately that she had a bluish discoloration on the outer part of her vagina. He took a biopsy and discovered carcinoma *in situ* of the vulva. He suggested surgery, since the disease was affecting a wide area. Moo was hospitalized for a week and within a month was again managing her large household.

She still travels with her husband. Twice a year, however, she returns for a complete gynecological exam, and with her she brings two large bags of fortune cookies made by one of her husband's companies.

"The cookies for my physician are special. I make certain the bakers always fill them with good fortunes, because it was my good fortune to find him." After seven years, she has had no recurrence of cancer.

Doris's story is more typical than Moo's of women with vulvar cancer. Although Doris has a private income, she works in a fashionable Los Angeles department store to finance her travels to exotic places.

Seven years ago she had some intolerable itching and discovered a raised lump of skin outside her vagina. She went to a physician who prescribed some cream to rub on it. The lump did not go away and the itching continued.

Doris went to another physician about a month later. He told her not to bother undressing; he knew exactly what she had and would prescribe one of the newest medications on the market.

Months later, still itching and burning, she found a third physician. This one seemed very concerned and told her that if the condition did not clear up in a few weeks to a month, he would do a biopsy. In the meantime, he assured her that she had nothing to worry about and gave her still another cream.

Doris was not satisfied. She wanted the lump biopsied. She called the director of a teaching hospital and found a specialist interested in diseases of the vulva, the area surrounding the external vaginal region. Her newest physician did the immediate biopsy she requested. The diagnosis: vulvar carcinoma.

Because there had been such a delay in treatment, Doris underwent very radical and disfiguring surgery. Most of the external vaginal area (the vulva) was removed. It took Doris a full month to recover physically and much longer to recover emotionally.

Today, however, if you were to question her about the surgery and its side effects, she would reply, "I am sixty-three years young. I still work. I still travel a great deal, and I still enjoy the company of some very interesting and attractive men. My life—and that includes my sex life—is a good one."

In 1981, the American Cancer Society estimates that there will be only about 4,500 new cases of vulvar cancer in the entire United States. Of these cases, between 500 and 1,000 will be fatal. It was noted from unpublished data of the Demographic Analysis Section, Biometry Branch, National Cancer Institute, that cancer of the vulva accounted for 0.3 percent of all female cancers, with a rate of 1.5 cases per 100,000 females. This means fewer than two women of every 100,000 will ever develop vulvar cancer. But for women over age fifty-five this is an important and unpublicized disease, and the risk goes up with each year of life.

THE VULVA

Vulva is a general term for the external parts of the female genital system. The name is given to the entire region surrounding the entrance to the vagina, out to the thighs and back to the rectum. The vagina is the canal that leads to the internal reproductive organs.

Long before birth, the structures of the vulva begin to become apparent. At three months in the womb, it is possible to differentiate between a male and a female fetus.

When a girl is born, her vulva is well developed, and it will not change much in appearance until she reaches puberty. Around the age of nine, ten, or eleven, hormonal changes will cause vulvar changes. The lips of the vagina will increase in size and hair will begin to grow.

The vulvar area is susceptible to problems as simple as an annoying case of vaginitis—an ordinary inflammation—and as complex as cancer. The common vulva vaginal problems affect thousands of women every day. Cancer in this area is very rare.

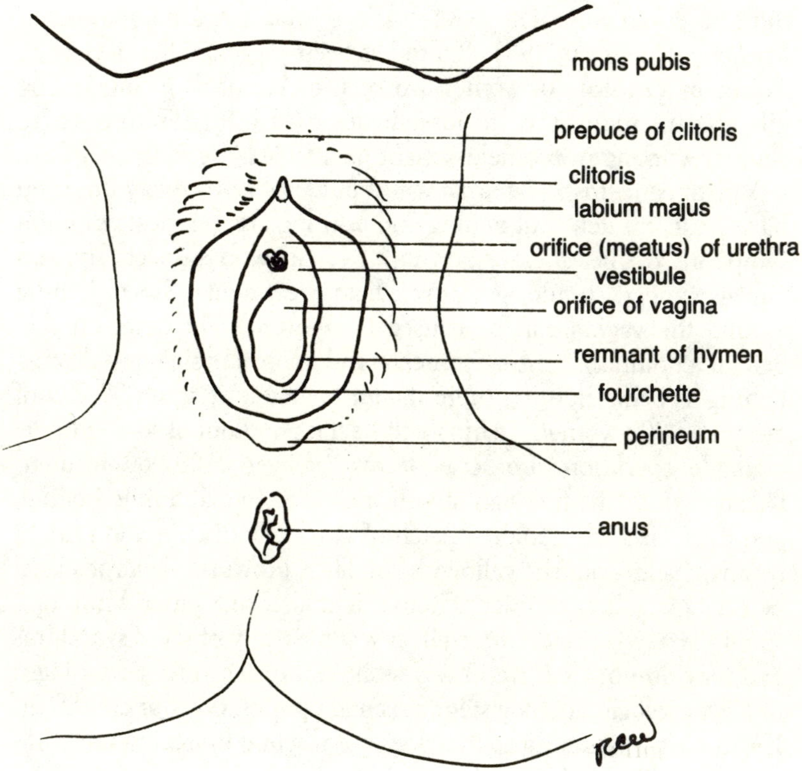

The anatomy of the vulva (the external part of the female genital system).

VULVAR CANCER AND ITS SYMPTOMS

It is extremely unlikely that a woman under the age of sixty will develop cancer of the vulva unless she had an early menopause. It is even more rare for any woman to develop vaginal cancer. Vulvar cancer appears to have no high-risk group, although some writers have suggested that women with herpetic lesions (see Chapter 10 on herpes) might have a higher incidence of this rare cancer. The most recent report of this was in *The New England Journal of Medicine*, August 6, 1981. It also has been suggested that it may be caused by exposure of women workers to chemicals in lubricating oils used in industry or to insecticides used in agriculture where women working in the fields might be affected.

Vulvar cancer is so rare that you should not worry every time you have a vaginal itch, but itching and burning are the most common symptoms of the disease, and any woman who suspects she has vulvar cancer should get immediate treatment. Since itching around the vagina can be caused by a number of other curable benign conditions, most women—and most physicians—dismiss itching as being nothing more than a bother. For about 99,999 of every 100,000 women, itching will be the symptom of some minor, treatable condition. For one or two of every 100,000 women, itching will be the first sign of vulvar cancer. In addition to itching, you might find a discolored patch of skin. The discoloration might be any shade—bluish, yellowish, pinkish, brownish—and it might be either vague or distinct. There might also be a raised lump or a small ulcer. To protect yourself, if you have any of these symptoms and they do not clear up in two weeks' time, see your gynecologist or a gynecologic oncologist for a second opinion on your condition. If you have a raised lump that does not respond to treatment within one week, have it biopsied.

In cases of very advanced vulvar cancer, you might have pain in the pelvic region and also some bleeding. These are usually symptoms associated with widespread disease.

An early form of vulvar cancer is called Bowen's Disease, or carcinoma *in situ* of the vulva. If you have this condition, the cure rate approaches 100 percent. Unfortunately, Bowen's Disease often has no symptoms. When it is caught, and cancer of the vulva is very rarely caught at this stage, it happens by chance. Usually during a routine exam an astute gynecologist will notice a discolored patch of skin or a slight change in skin texture. When this occurs, he or she will take a biopsy of the area, and within a few days the definitive diagnosis can be made.

The biopsy for carcinoma *in situ* or invasive vulvar cancer can be made with a dermatology punch or a scalpel blade. With a punch biopsy, a small instrument like the top of a fountain pen is pressed onto the area and a tiny circle of skin between 1/16 and 1/4 inch in diameter is withdrawn. This can be done in the physician's office. If your physician decides upon a scalpel blade, you might be hospitalized as an ambulatory patient.

It is unclear whether carcinoma *in situ* will progress to invasive cancer of the vulva if left alone, as can be the case with carcinoma *in situ* of the uterine cervix. By analogy, it is thought that cancer of the vulva probably will progress, too, at least in some cases.

If a biopsy proves positive, treatment for Bowen's Disease frequently involves surgery. Usually the skin is removed around the area where the cancerous tissues appear. Local applications of an anticancer drug—5 Florouracil (5FU)—also have been used with some degree of success for carcinoma *in situ;* this treatment is preferred to surgery by some physicians. *Cautery* or freezing techniques (discussed in Chapter 3 on the cervix) are being suggested as alternatives to surgery for this disease, but they have not yet become accepted methods at any of the major teaching centers. Some promising work is being done with the laser beam, however, its use is presently limited to some special research institutions.

Although cancer of the vulva is generally a very slow-growing disease and one that occurs in an area of the body that is easy to see and touch, most cases go undetected until the disease is already in the advanced stage. Why? Because most women over sixty today, who constitute the high-risk group, grew up in an era when "Don't touch yourself down there" was often heard. Women of this era (including many women now in their mid-thirties and forties) still shy away from touching the vaginal area. Routinely looking at themselves with a mirror is perhaps even more unusual among women in these age groups.

Physicians have been of little help to women with vaginal itches. Too often they simply say, "I'll give you some cream, and it will go away." Some physicians do not even bother having a woman with a vaginal or vulvar itch undress—and this is a disservice to their patients. If you have a vulvo-vaginal itch, insist on an examination. Esther's story will underline its importance.

Esther was an energetic woman in her early seventies living in fashionable Marin County, California. When she complained to her internist of some itching on her vulva, he did not examine her; he just gave her some hydrocortisone cream. The itching continued. A month later, the internist looked at the lesion and saw that there was a lump with a central ulcer. He referred Esther to a gynocologic oncologist, who performed a biopsy confirming his suspicion of invasive cancer of the vulva.

Because Esther had severe heart disease, her internist would not permit the recommended operation of a radical vulvectomy. She died from the disease nine months later—not having taken the chance that might have saved her.

Treating Vulvar Cancer

Treatment for invasive vulvar cancer is surgery, known as a radical vulvectomy and lymphadenectomy. This involves removal of the entire skin surface, the lips of the vagina, all the underlying fatty tissues, the regional lymph nodes in the groin area, and sometimes lymph nodes found deep in the pelvis. Lymph nodes are removed because malignant cells often travel to other parts of the body by way of the lymph system. The surgery is extensive and it often involves a full month's hospital stay. Because there is disfigurement, some surgeons may work with a plastic surgery team. Skin grafts, or the creation of special skin and muscle flaps, can be made when the skin has been removed. If you do develop this kind of cancer, you should try to find a gynecologic oncology team in a major teaching hospital and speak with good plastic surgeons before undergoing surgery.

While there is always an element of risk in surgery, the risks increase when the patient is in her sixties or older—the age group most vulnerable to vulvar cancer—and when the surgery is extensive. Because of its complexity and extent, the surgery itself sometimes proves fatal. Keep in mind, however, that despite the risks, there is a very good cure rate. Surgeons who treat the disease say that the cure rate is 85 percent if the cancer has not spread to the lymph nodes and 50 percent even if it has.

There are some alternatives to radical surgery, the most promising of which is a new, highly experimental freezing technique used at an Eastern European clinic and by several physicians in the United States.

Freezing requires special instruments and must be done in a hospital. It is not the same as routine office cryosurgery for warts or cervical dysplasia, which uses nitrous oxide or carbon dioxide. The advanced freezing technique for vulvar cancer uses cooling agents such as liquid nitrogen, followed by radiation to the lymph node-bearing area.

The benefits include no blood loss, almost no convalescence, less scarring, less pain. Why is it not used more extensively? The technique requires elaborate equipment and special skills. While freezing has been used effectively by physicians in other countries, physicians in America have not yet accomplished the results that are being accomplished in Europe. Even the physicians using the freezing technique admit that, in the long run, it may not be as effective as the standard treatment. Standard treatments have stood the test of time and are usually considered best. There are women, however, who feel that given the choices of extensive and painful surgery, an experimental technique that might buy time, and no treatment at all, the experimental freezing techniques might well be the best.

Radiation therapy is another alternative treatment for cancer of the vulva. The trouble is that there also are many reasons for *not* using radiation on this part of the body. The vulva is an easily contaminated area—hair bearing, moist, mobile, covered with clothes, and easily traumatized through sitting and rubbing. All these factors tend to offset the beneficial effects of radiation against the tumor and increase the misery and side effects suffered from the radiation treatment itself. The cure rate from radiation treatment is not as good as from surgery, and the complications may be severe and life threatening.

There are no dependable drugs for cancer of the vulva, although several have been used experimentally. Occasionally anticancer drugs are used for disease that has gone beyond the limits of surgical treatment.

Emotional Side Effects of Vulvar Surgery

What does a woman feel after a vulvectomy? We really do not know. Unlike breast surgery, vulvectomies are rare, and rarer still are the women who ever speak about it.

In the few instances when a young woman has a simple vulvectomy, chances are good that she will have some kind of cosmetic surgery. With support from friends, a lover, a professional therapist if needed, her emotional scars probably fade along with her surgical scars, particularly as she resumes her sex life.

In the past, physicians have often assumed that older women are so grateful to be alive that they care little about disfigurement. This seems hard to believe. It seems far more likely that these women have had no one to talk to about their experiences.

If you do develop this type of cancer, we suggest you check to see whether your hospital has a group such as I Can Cope or a liaison psychiatry team to help you with your emotional recovery. If your hospital does not have such a group or team, ask your surgeon to recommend a good psychotherapist or psychiatrist, preferably one with some experience in working with postsurgical patients.

RARE VARIATIONS ON CANCER OF THE VULVA

Pagets disease of the vulva is a bizarre type of disease that looks, under the microscope, like a form of cancer found in the nipple of a woman's breast. Its only symptom is an itchy reddish-white patch on the vulva that looks moist but is dry to the touch. Diagnosis is made by biopsy, and treatment is generally a wide local excision. If, in an even rarer instance, this disease is related to an underlying cancer of the sweat gland, a radical vulvectomy, sometimes followed by chemotherapy, is used.

Malignant melanoma of the vulva is basically a skin cancer on the vulva. It can affect women of any age. The symptom is a pigmented spot and definitive diagnosis is made by biopsy. The outlook for this type of disease generally is poor. Most physicians treat it with a radical vulvectomy. At centers in New York, Los Angeles, Houston, and Israel, however, immunotherapy is being used for this type of cancer. Since immunotherapy still is used only experimentally, it would be misleading to give statistics. The response rates differ from each of these centers. But you should not overlook this type of treatment. It is well worth comparing the statistics in terms of cure rates for immunotherapy and surgery at the various centers. To compare, ask the chief of staff to tell you how many patients were treated in the past five years with surgery and how many with surgery plus immunotherapy. Then ask the survival rate of each patient using each form of treatment to determine which treatment you will feel most comfortable using.

Nonmalignant Vulvar Diseases

There are myriad types of skin and venereal diseases of which women should be aware. Unless you are in your sixties you will not be concerned that these common problems might be cancerous. If you are in your sixties and have any kind of vulvo-vaginal problem, you should not be speculating; you should be seeking treatment. Most of these nonmalignant diseases are discussed fully in books such as *Our Bodies, Ourselves* and *My Body My Health: A Woman's Guide to Gynecology.*

The most common of these diseases is called herpes. It is of such importance that we have included a separate chapter on it. Herpes is not cancer. It is a vulvar disease that, ironically, is associated with cervical cancer.

Leukoplakia is another condition of which you should be aware. Leukoplakia is a white patch of skin found near mucus membranes of the vagina, anal region, and even the mouth. Many gynecologists say that leukoplakia is not a disease but a symptom. It may be Bowen's Disease (carcinoma *in situ)* or any of a number of benign conditions. The patch should always be biopsied to determine whether it is just an inflammation or cancer.

Can Vulvar Carcinoma Be Prevented?

To prevent a disease, one needs to know the cause of the disease. The cause of vulvar cancer is unknown. What can be prevented, however, is the spread of the disease. Early detection is the key. Because the symptoms of vulvar cancer so resemble common itching problems, half the women with vulvar cancer experience a delay of almost six months between the time they first notice the symptoms and their diagnosis. You should insist upon a biopsy of any lump or sore that is treated, but does not regress or clear up within one or two weeks.

VAGINAL CANCER

Cancer of the vagina, excluding cancer associated with DES (see Chapter 4), is even rarer than vulvar cancer. Fewer than 0.6 per 100,000 women will ever develop this disease, and less than 350 women now alive in the United States will die of cancer of the vagina. There are several kinds of vaginal malignancies. They include:

Dysplasia of the vagina This is very similar to dysplasia of the cervix, although it is very unusual and rarely seen and may not have the same premalignant potential as dysplasia of the cervix.

Carcinoma *in situ* of the vagina This is just like carcinoma *in situ* of the cervix; only the location is different.

Squamous carcinoma or cancer of the vagina This is very rarely encountered. When it occurs, it generally is in women over the age of sixty-five.

Vaginal and cervical cancers actually can be the same type of cancer. Carcinoma *in situ* and cancer of the vagina occasionally occur in women who have already been successfully treated for cancer of the cervix, suggesting that the same agent or agents has then begun to work on the vagina. The only symptoms of vaginal malignancies are bleeding and discharge.

Treatment of cancer of the vagina is similar to treatment of cancer of the cervix. Either surgery or radiation may be used, separately or occasionally in combination.

Nonmalignant Vaginal Conditions: Cystoceles and Rectoceles

Some women are aware of a bulge inside the vagina; it may even protrude outside the vagina. Such bulges may be due to cystoceles or rectoceles. These are, respectively, protrusions and descents of the anterior and posterior vaginal wall and are often the result of a long and difficult childbirth, which weakens the vaginal walls. They are sometimes associated with the problems of a leaky bladder. The cervix and uterus also may hang down and protrude when their supports are likewise weakened.

Although women in their thirties may have this type of problem, it is far more frequent after menopause. Involuntary loss of urine associated with cystoceles is sometimes controlled with modest weight loss and simple exercises. If surgery is advised for cystocele or rectocele and you are in your thirties, get a second opinion!

Bulges and protrusions of this sort are not indicative of cancer of the genital tract except in the most unusual cases. Once in a great while these will be brought on by increased abdominal pressure due to malignant disease elswhere, especially in the intestinal tract. The discerning physician will investigate the possibility of cancer elsewhere before trying to relieve the symptoms caused by these bulges.

Chapter Ten

The Herpes Epidemic, Cancer, and You

Pia was at boarding school when she discovered a small itchy sore near her vagina. Actually it consisted of not one but several small tender blisters. Her friends suggested she pack her vagina with yogurt, a popular home remedy. When this didn't work, she went to the school infirmary where the nurse gave her a medicated cream. The cream seemed to work, and the sores disappeared.

Three months later Pia had a recurrence of the sores. She went home, and her sister took her to a gynecologist who had a laboratory test done to determine their nature. Diagnosis: herpes virus; in Pia's case, transmitted through sexual intercourse.

Estimates are that as many as 5 million American men and women have herpes in an active or dormant state.

Herpes, which is affecting more women today than ever before, is one of the most annoying and enigmatic diseases known. No one seems to know very much about it, and, what is most disheartening, it is barely treatable and not curable. Classified as a vulvar disease, it has been identified as cancer-related, but paradoxically its main association has been with cervical cancer, not vulvar cancer.

Because genital herpes usually is transmitted through sexual intercourse, it is commonly called the love virus, and medical researchers classify it as a venereal disease. As with other venereal diseases, the incidence of herpes seems to be increasing among people of all social classes, according to studies by William Rollo of McMahon University in Ontario, on the epidemiology of herpes. The disease is a serious problem in the United States today.

There are a number of different types of herpes infections, some associated with mononucleosis and some associated with chicken pox and shingles. HVH-1 is herpes virus hominis or herpes simplex virus (HSV-1), the type that is generally associated with cold sores on the mouth. This is not generally considered a venereal disease. Herpes simplex 2 or herpes virus hominis (HVH-2) is genital herpes, and it is most often associated with sores on the vulva, the outside of the vagina. It is this genital herpes virus that women should try to avoid.

The two forms are interchangeable in location. "Physicians today are seeing more HSV-1 in the genital regions and HSV-2 in the mouth regions," says Dr. Priscilla Schaffer. Dr. Schaffer is working on herpes virus research; she is associate professor of microbiology and molecular genetics at the Sidney Farber Cancer Institute, Harvard Medical School.

Dr. Schaffer says that the interchange of the two forms of herpes seems to be the result of our society's greater practice of oral-genital sex. It is theoretically possible and highly likely that this virus is passed not just from men to women and vice versa, but from women to women, from men to men, from men to women to men, or any other variation. (In homosexual males, the virus is also found around the anal area.)

While there is no evidence to support anyone who tries to blame a case of herpes on the proverbial toilet seat rather than on sexual intercourse, Dr. Schaffer noted that it really isn't clear from the nature of the virus that sexual intercourse is the *only* means of transmission.

It has been suggested that current clothing fashions may contribute to the severity of herpes, though they do not *cause* the disease itself. Dr. Robert E. Hardy, a Greenwich, Connecticut, obstetrician who frequently treats genital herpes, has said that he and many of his colleagues feel the combination of tight-fitting jeans and nylon panties are aggravating herpes. The tightness of the clothes irritates the vulva terribly, while the synthetic fabric of nylon panties prevents moisture from escaping, according to Dr. Hardy. The combination is something the skin just cannot tolerate, he says, and it makes an ideal milieu in which herpes can flourish. But the virus itself actually lives in the nerves which go to the skin.

SYMPTOMS AND TREATMENT

The herpes sores or ulcers are the most obvious symptoms of the disease. They look like chancre sores or blisters, and they appear within two to seven days after exposure to the disease. Other symptoms may include a burning sensation during urination, fever, and chills.

To be certain the sores are those of herpes, you will need confirmation by a physician. The physician usually will take a cotton swab and get a sample of fluid from the sores. The fluid can be rubbed across a glass slide and analyzed under a microscope, or the virus can be grown in a laboratory culture.

The initial attack of herpes usually is the strongest. There is no cure for the disease, and it will never entirely go away. This is because the herpes virus is not like other viruses, such as German measles (rubella). If you have had German measles once, you will never get it again. You develop antibodies against it. An antibody is a protein substance developed by the body to neutralize the invading virus, and the antibodies remain in the body after the first attack to defend it against any subsequent ones. Some antibodies diminish within the body over a period of time, which is why you can catch some diseases more than once, but those for German measles do not do so appreciably. It is for this reason that a vaccination for German measles confers permanent immunity against the disease.

With genital herpes, however, an unusual thing happens: The virus lives within the cells in the nervous system, where antibodies—which are carried by the bloodstream—cannot get to it. Thus the antibody defense system will not prevent recurring attacks; the virus can always travel by the nerve in which it lives to the skin surface, where it will form new lesions. Some women, and some physicians, have speculated that since the virus lives in the nervous system, new attacks may be brought on by stress. There is no solid evidence for this, but if you ask any woman what happens to her when she is going through "a bad time," chances are she will answer, "When my nerves are on end, this damned infection is worse than ever. I don't care what the studies say!"

Herpes may be contagious *even when sores are not detectible* and the disease seems to be in a quiescent (dormant) state. It is especially dangerous to infants, who may be infected in the process of being born. For example, a 1980 study of herpes-afflicted infants showed that 70 percent of the mothers had no symptoms of the virus in their genital systems. Because herpes infections can be fatal to the newborn, cesarean deliveries are indicated for women who have the disease.

Genital herpes also is worrisome because of its association with cervical cancer. This does not appear to be a case of cause-and-effect, rather, it is a statistical association: Women who have had carcinoma *in situ* of the cervix or invasive cervical cancer tend to have herpes antibodies in their blood more often than women who have not had cervical cancer. It may be that herpes is "a fellow traveler"—not the cause of cancer but related to the cause.

However, there is one bit of disturbing evidence regarding herpes and cancer. "While the statistical association between HSV-2 and human cancer is stronger than that of HSV-1, normal cells are changed into cancerous ones from both Type I and Type 2 virus," said Dr. Schaffer. "I do want to stress, however, that this has taken place in cell cultures only and may not be happening in humans. The possibility exists, however," she added.

The Treatment for Herpes

Although herpes is to some degree treatable, there is no effective cure and most treatments do not seem to alleviate the problem very well. Attempts have been made to deactivate herpes with special dyes that accept light energy that will break up the virus. The problem with this photoinactivation technique is that it may, in itself, predispose you to cancer. Do not accept this as treatment. Other direct chemical applications to control the virus include the use of ether and similar chemical agents, but these are frequently quite painful. Ether has another drawback: It is explosive.

Experimental work with the use of lysine, an amino acid that is a normal food constituent, suggested improved control of herpetic infection, but recent studies show that lysine is not the answer.

Wet compresses on the sores as well as sitz baths will help slightly. Some physicians report success with laser therapy, but this is not generally recommended.

Dr. Schaffer thinks women should be aware of a new treatment that at the time of this writing was just being used in clinical trials; it is a drug called acyclovir. From the laboratory studies it appears to be a promising new antiherpes drug.

PREVENTION IS BEST

Perhaps the best answer to controlling herpes is prevention. If a man with whom you are having sex has herpes, insist that he use a condom. For six to eight weeks after his initial attack of herpes, *he could still be contagious*. Remember that even in the absence of open sores, a person with the virus may transmit it to another person.

Do not have intercourse at all if your sexual partner has active open sores; also avoid oral sex. If a man with whom you are having sex has herpes, he will suffer, but you will have the more serious symptoms. Herpes is treatable, but not curable. If you develop herpes, you will have it the rest of your life. Knowing your sexual partner more than just casually may help you from contracting herpes.

The American Social Health Association has formed a national group called HELP that can give up-to-date information about herpes and treatment progress reports. There is a small membership fee. To contact the organization write to HELP, Box 100, Palo Alto, California 94302.

Chapter Eleven

Treatment: New Hope For Cancer Patients

The main treatments for cancer today are surgery, chemotherapy, radiation, and combinations of the three. Despite the new openness in discussing cancer, many people still have difficulty bringing themselves to talk about the details of these treatments and their side effects. This is hardly surprising. Surgery always carries some element of risk, and the side effects of chemotherapy and radiation are not pleasant. Still, it is necessary to know these things if you are to make intelligent decisions about yourself—about what risks and pains are worth accepting—or to understand what other people are going through. We cannot emphasize too strongly that many women are alive today because they persevered with these treatments despite all risks and side effects. Also, researchers and physicians are continually finding new ways to improve surgical techniques and to minimize the discomfort caused by drugs and radiation.

Where the chapters on specific cancers discuss the various treatments for that particular cancer, this chapter presents an overview of the traditional forms of treatment and the side effects that most concern women. In addition, it includes some of the newer forms of therapy being explored in the search for the elusive magic bullet—the cure for cancer.

WHAT TO EXPECT FROM SURGERY: BEFORE AND AFTER

Of the forms of treatment for cancer, surgery is usually the primary one, particularly in gynecological cancers. It is only with choriocarcinoma, a cancer rare in the United States that mimics pregnancy, that chemotherapy is considered a first-choice treatment. In some very early cases of breast cancer, radiation *might* be an alternative treatment of choice.

By the time a person is operated on for cancer, malignant cells have formed solid masses visible to the naked eye, and it is possible for the surgeon to cut them out. Usually surrounding tissues are also removed as a precautionary measure.

Except in cases of breast, vaginal, and vulvar cancer, the actual surgery for most types of female cancer will be a variation of the standard hysterectomy. In the United States today, two types of hysterectomies are performed. They are called abdominal and vaginal, depending on where the initial incision is made. Usually in cases of cancer of the reproductive tract, the surgeon will perform an abdominal hysterectomy. This procedure gives the doctor a better view of the surrounding organs. For the same reason, the surgeon usually uses the old-fashioned longitudinal cut up and down the abdomen, rather than the bikini cut across the top of the pubic hairline. The latter, which results in a less visible scar, is used for hysterectomies when no cancer is involved and—in an unrelated instance—for cesarean deliveries.

Whatever the form of surgery, the preliminaries will be much the same for the patient upon entering the hospital. Your physician will begin by ordering a number of tests, including the following:

Blood type and blood count The first is to determine your blood type, so that the right kind of blood will be ready in the event you need a transfusion; the second is intended to tell the surgical team whether or not you are anemic or suffering from infection, in which case they might want to defer the operation.

Urinalysis This is a check on your general health, since much can be told about the body's organs from the different materials that are excreted in the urine.

Electrocardiogram (EKG) This determines whether or not you have any heart problems—important information for the anesthesiologist as well as the surgeon.

Special procedures Depending on the type of surgery you receive, you will probably have an x-ray to be certain your lungs are clear. X-rays of the urinary system and bowels are frequently useful in planning surgery. Cystoscopy (looking into the bladder) and sigmoidoscopy or colonoscopy (looking into the intestine) are necessary before treating many types of cancer. Because procedures must be individualized, ask your physician to spell out to you in detail all the preliminary tests that he or she is ordering and why they are necessary.

The day before surgery, your doctor will make arrangements for you to talk to the anesthesiologist if you have not done so already. It is important that you know who this person is and that he or she knows who you are. In recent years the role of the anesthesiologist has been expanding. As medical writer Laurence Cherry noted in a *New York Times Magazine* article of June 3, 1979: "Far from merely putting patients to sleep, anesthesiologists today are really the physicians in charge of patients during surgery as well as supervision of special care and pain relief afterwards."

You should find out what drugs the anesthesiologist intends to use and what their side effects are, so that you will know what to expect after the operation. If a particular pain killer doesn't work very well for you, if you think you are allergic to a particular drug, you want to be very sure that the anesthesiologist knows about it.

The evening before surgery you probably will be given an enema. You also will be "prepped"—that is, prepared for surgery.

In the case of a hysterectomy or vaginal surgery, your pubic hair may be shaved although some surgeons shave only immediately before surgery; some doctors may also order a douche. In breast surgery, the procedure differs slightly.

Before going to the operating room, you will be given an injection. This will help you relax and make you feel somewhat sleepy, but you will still be alert enough to recognize the surgeon. Then the anesthesiologist will step in (Most hysterectomies in the United States are done under general anesthesia). Barbiturates are very useful for inducing sleep and are frequently used. Curare or one of its synthetic derivatives also may be given intraveneously in order to relax your muscles; this is especially helpful in abdominal surgery, since the stomach muscles retain their tension despite the general anesthetic.

Since most of the muscle relaxants also prevent spontaneous breathing, the anesthesiologist will use a mechanical respirator to keep your lungs working. Generally a mask will be put over your face so that you can inhale a special combination of nitrous oxide and other gases. As an aid to breathing, a tube may also be inserted into your mouth and down to your windpipe.

At the conclusion of the operation, the anesthesiologist will use still other drugs to reverse the effect of the muscle relaxants, thus enabling you to breathe again on your own.

Each of the drugs used by the anesthesiologist has its own advantages, hazards, and side effects. In a small percentage of cases, some gases will have toxic side effects on the kidneys, liver, or other organs. Many combinations of the different anesthetic agents also leave some women with nausea and weakness. In addition, many women complain of having a stiff neck following anesthesia, because of the positioning of the head to permit the passage of the tube into the windpipe. These are all matters to discuss in advance with the anesthesiologist. If you have a competent anesthesiologist, you need not go into surgery worrying about its side effects.

As for surgery itself, the most common side effects today are wound infection, pneumonia, urinary tract infections, and anemia. If the abdomen doesn't heal properly hernias may also develop, although they can occur if the surgeon does not close the wound securely enough. A hernia is a weak spot in the abdominal wall where an organ such as the intestine can push forward because of internal pressure. It is common in cancer patients who have had surgery and particularly in women who are markedly overweight or have serious dietary deficiencies. One way surgeons are attempting to prevent complications is by using plastic or stainless steel wires for "retention" sutures, which can be removed after healing is completed. Women who are very thin sometimes find them to be uncomfortable. If you are thin, be sure to ask your surgeon whether there is an alternative in your particular case.

The best protection against anything going wrong is to select a surgeon who does the kind of surgery you need on a routine basis. The best way to find out how often a surgeon is involved with cancer cases of a particular type is to ask. The individual chapters of this book give some idea of how often the various kinds of surgery are done. Keep the physician's specialty in perspective. Since vulvar and vaginal cancer affect only 5,000 women in the United States each year, a surgeon who treats only a few women per year might be considered an expert. Breast cancer, on the other hand, affects 100,000 women, and a surgeon who does breast surgery only a few times per month might not be the best.

Today most physicians treating cancer patients work in teams. It is crucial that you have a good rapport with your physician, not only for your peace of mind but also for discussing your treatment—and your follow-up treatments, should they be necessary. You will want to know what to expect from these. You will also want an honest evaluation of what to expect should you refuse follow-up treatment.

CHEMOTHERAPY AND ITS SIDE EFFECTS

Chemotherapy is the use of drugs for the treatment and control of disease. While any disease can be treated this way, the term today usually refers to cancer treatment. The idea of using chemotherapy in cancer cases was developed some thirty years ago as part of the physician's master plan: First the physician would attack cancer with the knife, removing the tumor through surgery. Then drugs would be deployed throughout the body on what amounted to search-and-destroy missions. The hope was that they would travel throughout the body, finding and killing cancer cells that had been missed by the knife. Frequently the plan worked.

The aim of chemotherapy is either to completely destroy the cancer cell or in some way to interfere with the cell's ability to reproduce. It is believed that cancer drugs alter the cancer cell's genetic composition in such a way that they halt the cell's ability to divide and replicate and survive.

Different families of drugs are used in chemotherapy treatment. Some are highly toxic metal substances, some are related to gases used during wars, but some are actually from natural plants. The drugs most often used for treatment in female cancers are listed on the following chart:

Common Name	Other Names	Type of Cancer Treated
Alkylating agents		
Chlorambucil	Leukeran	Breast and ovarian
Cyclophosphamide	Endoxan, Cytoxan	Breast and ovarian
Nitrogen mustard	HN2, Mustargen, Mechlorethamine	Breast and ovarian
Phenylalanine mustard	L-Sarcolysin, Melphalan, Alkeran	Breast and ovarian
Thio TEPA	TSPA	
Triethylene melamine	TEM	

Common Name	Other Names	Type of Cancer Treated
Antimetabolites		
5-fluorouracil	5-FU	Breast and ovarian
6-mercaptopurine	6-MP, Purinethol	Choriocarcinoma
Mexthotrexate	Amethopterin	Breast and choriocarcinoma
Mitotic Inhibitors		
Vinblastine sulfate	Velban	Breast and choriocarcinoma
Vincristine sulfate	Oncovin	Breast
Antibiotics & Related substances		
Actinomycin D	Dactinomycin, Cosmegen, Meractinomycin	Breast
Adriamycin		Ovary, sarcoma
Random Synthetics		
Cis-platinum	Cis-dichlorodiammine platinum, DDP	Ovarian
Hormonal agents		
Progesterone Megace Depo-Provera		Endometrial

(A variety of hormone compounds are used in breast cancer therapy, most often in cases of metastases.)

Chemotherapy is given in a number of ways. The most common include oral doses as a liquid or pill, direct injection into a muscle or vein, intravenous drip, and injection into an artery or directly into the abdomen.

The way a particular drug is administered often depends on the type of cancer being treated. Chemotherapy is not a generalized treatment; it must be tailored to meet each patient's needs. Be certain to ask the physician or the nurse administering treatment how the drugs will be given, what side effects you might expect, how you might minimize the side effects, and how long your course of treatment will be. Because the side effects of chemotherapy can be so serious, chemotherapy has acquired a bad name. Some women still say that if they ever develop cancer, they would never consent to being "poisoned" by a chemical. This attitude is counterproductive. Side effects do occur, but most are reversible. It is, however, of great importance that you find physicians skilled in the use of modern effective chemotherapy.

In gynecological cancers, physicians or specially trained nurses might administer chemotherapy. Those most experienced will probably be involved in giving ten to twenty treatments to various patients per week.

The most serious side effect of chemotherapy is the suppression of bone marrow production. The bone marrow cells are responsible for production of white and red blood cells. Anticancer drugs may also affect the liver and kidneys. To protect against serious side effects, your physician will perform special blood tests to determine how the anticancer drugs are affecting you.

A temporary neurologic side effect is a numbing or tingling sensation in the arms or legs. This occurs because the drugs sometimes affect the nervous system.

Hair loss has been called one of the most distressing side effects of chemotherapy. Substantial hair loss, however, may be prevented by cooling the scalp. Ice bonnets are available in many hospitals today. If you do not have one at your hospital, bring ice packs for your treatments. Place them on your head about fifteen minutes before treatment and keep them there for about thirty to forty-five minutes after treatment. Be careful not to freeze your skin, especially your ears. Remember, too, that with or without ice bonnets, not all women experience hair loss.

Nausea and vomiting also occur frequently. In some cases they are due to irritation of the lining of the stomach or the intestines; in other cases, the drugs trigger parts of the brain to cause nausea and vomiting. Many different ways of forestalling and alleviating nausea and vomiting have been tried, including the use of sedatives, intravenous fluids, visualization therapy, and marijuana. Compazine, thorazine, torecan, tigan, and dramamine are among the medications that have been tried, all with varying degrees of effectiveness, dependability, and predictability. Droperidol, a potent tranquilizer, does prevent or reduce nausea, but it is difficult to use outside an operating room where special supportive equipment is available. Morphine, meperidine, and similar narcotic agents frequently will allay the urge to vomit, but they have other unwanted side effects such as respiratory depression.

Today marijuana is widely thought to be an effective means of controlling nausea due to chemotherapy. Some patients find that smoking marijuana or, preferably, eating it produces a marked improvement in their ability to tolerate drug-induced nausea. It is the active ingredient of marijuana, tetrahydrocannabinol, commonly known as THC, that appears to be so effective in reducing the nausea and vomiting related to chemotherapy. The effect has been documented in many studies, including one at Duke University Medical Center in early 1980. By June 1980 the Food and Drug Administration noted that THC in pill or capsule form—already used by government researchers—could be made available to some 4,000 physicians at cancer centers treating patients with chemotherapy.

A basic book on the subject is *Using Marijuana in the Reduction of Nausea Associated with Chemotherapy* by Roger A. Rothman, assistant professor of social work at the University of Washington, where he is also division head for research training at the University's Alcoholism and Drug Abuse Institute (see the book list at the end of this chapter). Besides describing the psychological and physiological effects of marijuana, Professor Rothman also discusses ways of acquiring, preparing, and using it. He even gives some recipes for including marijuana in foods. In addition, the laws governing marijuana are covered.

According to Professor Rothman, smoking marijuana will bring relief from nausea within five to ten minutes, and the effect will last about two hours. If mixed with food or put into capsules and swallowed, marijuana takes longer to bring relief (forty-five minutes to two hours), but the effect also tends to last longer—two to six hours. Finally, Professor Rothman notes that if the idea of smoking is abhorrent, or if the nausea is so severe that eating is impossible, marijuana can be taken in suppository form; in that case, relief will come in about thirty minutes, and the effect will last about two hours.

Marijuana, like more conventional drugs, does not work for everyone. Not everyone gets high on marijuana either. Still, it has been a great boon to many cancer patients. One young mother who finally started using marijuana at the suggestion of her physician after other drugs had failed, put it this way: "With marijuana, I knew I could depend on its working for me. When I was trying different medication and shots every week, it was 'God, I hope it's going to work.' Sometimes it did, for a few treatments; then it might not work. Every few weeks the doctor would say, 'This time I've got it. You'll be fine.' Then I would go home and throw up for three hours. Once I was on marijuana, that was it. I was fine during the full year of chemotherapy."

New drugs are still being studied to combat nausea—metoclopramide is the most recent—and many physicians say the drugs will eventually outweigh marijuana's effectiveness.

To cope with the loss of appetite and nausea so common among patients receiving chemotherapy and radiation, a booklet called "Nutrition for the Cancer Patient" has been prepared by the U.S. Department of Health, Education, and Welfare. This is an annotated bibliography that includes diet guides, food tips, and special diets. (A listing of the individual booklets is in the bibliography at the end of this chapter.)

Some suggestions regarding diet and/or nausea from treatments include:

- Eat salty foods rather than sweet ones.
- Suck on flavored ice cubes made from fruit juices.
- Try to walk around after eating rather than napping immediately.

To help ease yourself into eating on a regular diet plan:

- Eat mini meals throughout the day.
- Drink milk shakes with added powdered milk.
- Eat yogurt.
- Drink through a straw—slowly.
- For nutritious foods such as vegetables and even meats that you don't feel like chewing, strain and use in soups.

If the smell of food makes you sick, ask someone else to prepare it; then, on your good days, make several meals in advance and freeze them.

Always remember the importance of eating well-balanced meals, no matter how unappetizing the mere thought of food is, let alone the food itself. The body needs all the energy it can get to make up for the drain imposed by the disease, weight loss, and treatments.

The way you react to chemotherapy may also depend upon your psychological state. Dr. Bernard S. Siegel, assistant clinical professor of surgery at the Yale University School of Medicine, believes that many women suffer loss of appetite and nausea as a result of chemotherapy because their physicians have unknowingly encouraged such negative reactions. When a physician says, in effect, "This is poison; it will make you sick," many women dutifully follow their doctor's suggestion and proceed to get sick, according to Dr. Siegel.

It also appears that women who do not like their doctors, or who do not really have faith in the efficiency of the treatment they are getting, tend to become sicker than those who are involved in a working partnership with their physicians. Sometimes women have stopped vomiting from chemotherapy just by changing doctors. Most often it is when women (and men, too, for that matter) view chemotherapy as something positive that positive changes occur within them.

"A woman who sees chemotherapy as life saving, as the nectar of the gods, will fare much better than a woman who sees it as a poison," says Dr. Siegel. "She will in many cases receive treatment and—without nausea, vomiting, or loss of appetite—go off to be with her family and friends or resume work. Why is this possible? Because she believes she is being made well."

RADIATION THERAPY AND ITS SIDE EFFECTS

The other common form of cancer treatment is radiation therapy, also called radiotherapy, x-ray therapy, irradiation, radiation treatment, and cobalt treatment. Radiation therapy is simply the controlled emission of high-energy rays. When used against a tumor, radiation kills the cancer cells or interferes with their ability to reproduce, and the tumor shrinks in size.

There are two ways that radiation is administered today: externally (teletherapy), which is the most common method; and internally (brachytherapy). In internal radiation, tiny implants filled with radioactive materials are placed inside the body, sometimes directly into tumors. These usually are left in place for a few days. Internal radiation is used in the treatment of cervical cancer and is fully explained in Chapter 3.

With external radiation, different units are used with different energy sources. Some machines have a radioactive substance such as cobalt inside them. As the material decays, it emits radiation that is harnessed for treatment. Other units such as linear accelerators or betatrons are able to create their own energy. The machines are large, awesome-looking units—rectangular boxes perhaps eight by ten feet in size. Some have rotating hoods that can be directed over a tumor area, and some have special "eyes" that can focus onto the tumor from a distance. The type of machine and the radiation dosage used depend upon the size and location of the tumor, as well as the availability of the devices. Smaller hospitals may have just one unit.

Radiation therapy is usually administered at hospitals, although some communities have radiation therapists who work from offices. Because radiation therapy is so specialized a field, it is important that anyone receiving such treatment go to a center where it is administered by a person specially trained and certified in therapeutic radiation (as opposed to diagnostic x-ray radiation). This person will be thoroughly experienced in knowing what dosages to give and how to give the maximum dosage to tumors with minimal damage to normal cells.

Should radiation treatments be necessary, you will meet with a radiotherapist before receiving treatment. At this time you might undergo x-rays to determine the exact size of the tumor and its location. Then the tumor's position will be marked with ink so the operator of the radiation unit will know exactly where to direct the radiation. You should be sure not to wash off the marks until treatments are completed. The number of treatments will vary depending upon the tumor. Usually they will be given over a period of four to five weeks, typically in many short sessions.

Radiation treatments are given in a special room that in many centers today is cheerfully decorated. You might sit in a chair or lie on a tablelike surface. Probably you will see nothing more than a large box with a rotating hood. Special shields might be placed over parts of your body to protect you from excess radiation. Some of the newer machines, however, have a built-in protection device.

Not surprisingly, people are usually nervous about radiation treatments. Many stories about the side effects of radiation harken back to the old days of radiation burns and severe nausea. Today, even with newer and safer units, women still worry. According to Dr. Rita Girolamo, professor of radiology at New York Medical College, the single most common question is the simple one, "Will it hurt?" The answer to this is no, says Dr. Girolamo. However, you can expect side effects, perhaps including a suntanned look and a roughness in the area being treated. Hair loss, which concerns many women, only occurs in the area receiving radiation. Other side effects may include nausea, fatigue, and diarrhea. These may not appear until the fourth or fifth day after treatment begins or possibly later.

To control nausea, marijuana might be effective, and its use is discussed in the preceding section on chemotherapy. To control diarrhea you may talk with your physician about changing your diet gradually to include high-bulk foods such as bananas, apple sauce, and white rice (not brown). Sometimes boiled milk is effective; however, it must be boiled for a full five minutes. Other suggestions about diet are included in a booklet prepared by the National Cancer Institute called "Radiation Therapy and You: A Guide to Self-Help During Treatment."

More serious side effects can include ulceration of the rectum and large intestine and diminished capacity of the bladder to hold urine. If you are working with a highly skilled radiation team that has access to sophisticated new equipment, you probably have less to worry about. You should, however, ask what side effects you can expect.

In addition to asking about side effects, be certain you understand just how long treatment might continue, whom you will be treated by, and whom you can call if you have any questions—day or night.

OTHER NEW TREATMENTS

In addition to surgery, chemotherapy, and radiation, physicians are experimenting with other forms of treatment for cancer. These range from immunotherapy—the use of an outside agent to stimulate the body's natural defense system—to a return to the century-old practice of heat therapy, or hyperthemia, a superheating of the body's tissues. The principal new treatments include the following:

Immunotherapy Three methods of immunotherapy are being used today, all of which have shown some promise for treating metastic disease, particularly breast cancers. In *active immunotherapy*, modified tumor cells—that is, cells that have been altered by radiation, enzymes, or other techniques—are used to stimulate heightened anticancer response from the patient's body. *Passive immunotherapy* is an experimental method of harvesting anticancer antibodies from one individual and using them to fight cancer in another. Finally there is *adjuvant or nonspecific immunotherapy*, which involves the use of substances like BCG, an extract from tuberculosis-type bacteria. This is injected into a patient in an attempt to trigger anticancer mechanisms. There is nothing wrong with immunotherapy in principle, but it has not always achieved the most desirable results in practice. Since it is generally without serious side effects, women can look to it as a new promise, a new hope.

Interferon Possibly the most important agent in stimulating the body's immune system, interferon is a natural protetin that all bodies have. It can fight viruses and cancer. The cost of interferon has been so astronomical and the supply so limited that it did not seem practical for treatment until recently. In 1980 a miraculous breakthrough occurred. A team of scientists found a method of planting a human gene in a bacteria substance that eventually produced interferon. As a result, interferon is now being manufactured by pharmaceutical firms. Initial work for treatment of some female cancers looks hopeful. However, much more needs to be learned; this is not the "magic bullet." You should consult with your physician or the National Cancer Institute to determine whether interferon might be useful in your particular case. To date, the publicity for interferon is far ahead of its known usefulness, especially in treatment of female cancers.

Photoradiation Now under study at the Roswell Park Memorial Hospital in Buffalo, New York, photoradiation is one of the newest experimental techniques. For this treatment a patient is given a photoactive (activated by light) material intravenously. The material accumulates in the tumor area as well as in various surrounding tissues. Several days later, by using a special red light delivered from a laser, the material is activated in what researchers call an excited form of oxygen, which eventually has a lethal effect on the tumor cells' membranes.

Hyperthermia The treatment of disease by inducing a high fever dates back to the 1890s when Dr. William Coley injected cancer patients with cultures of a killed virus—"Coley's mixed toxins," as these killed cultures came to be called. These produced certain features of normal bacterial infections, including high fever, and in a substantial number of cases the tumors regressed.

Hyperthermia is still used today. Immersing the patient in hot-water baths appears to increase the effectiveness of chemotherapy and radiation. Whole-body hyperthermia also is being studied as a means of effecting a cancer remission in cases of metastitic disease. The original studies were done at the National Cancer Institute under senior investigator Dr. Joan Bull.

Lipid Vesicles Still very much in the experimental stage, these are microscopic capsules with a fatty (lipid) encasement. Lipid vesicles are intended to deliver chemotherapy drugs such as methotrexate directly to the tumor. The aim is to reduce harmful side effects on the rest of the body by bypassing other tissues. The vesicles work in two ways. In the first, local hyperthermia is used to heat the cancer site. Then the vesicles are injected into the body. They follow the bloodstream to the tumor, where the heat disintegrates their encasement, thus releasing the drug at just the right place. In the second method an antigen (a substance that activates the immune response of normal cells) is placed on the surface of the vesicles. This puts the normal cells on their guard, so to speak, as the vesicle passes by, en route to the tumor site.

Vitamin C and Laetrile These controversial substances are not new, nor are they a part of traditional treatments, but pressure from supporters has resulted in their being tested at major cancer centers.

Discovered in the late 1920s by Albert Szent-Gyorgi, vitamin C was popularized in the 1970s as a treatment for the common cold by Linus Pauling, a Nobel Prize winner in chemistry and in peace. After other investigators reported that cancer patients had unusually low reserves of ascorbate (the salt of ascorbic acid, or vitamin C), Pauling and a Scottish associate, Dr. Ewan Cameron, theorized this was not due simply to poor nutrition but to an increased utilization of—and need for—the vitamin. While conceding that further research had to be done, especially in chemotherapy cases (Cameron's studies of vitamin C in Scotland had not included anyone receiving chemotherapy), Pauling suggested that all cancer patients receive a minimum dose of ten grams of vitamin C a day. This should be given consistently, he emphasized.

No evidence to support the Pauling-Cameron theory was found

when vitamin C was tested at the Comprehensive Cancer Center of the Mayo Clinic. Said Dr. Charles Moertel, director of the center and chairman of its department of oncology, "It didn't work. I wish it did, but it didn't."

Some 140 advanced cancer patients, for whom no other treatment was effective, participated in the Mayo Clinic study. Half the group received vitamin C and half the group received a placebo in its stead. It was a double-blind study, meaning that neither the patients nor the people administering the doses to them knew who was receiving vitamin C and who was receiving placebos until after the investigation was concluded. "When we broke the code," said Dr. Moertel, "there was no significant difference between those who took the placebos and those who took the vitamin C."

The Mayo study was not strictly comparable to Cameron's, since the American patients had received chemotherapy and radiation treatments while the Scottish ones had not. Because of this difference, Pauling asserted that the Mayo test did not invalidate Cameron's work. For his part, Moertel conceded that a different group of patients might have produced a different result. But he noted an immense practical difficulty: "When you know that chemotherapy might effect a cure in someone, you are not going to say, 'Don't take this known cure, but take vitamin C instead.' That would be totally irresponsible."

Still more controversial than vitamin C is laetrile, an extract of apricot pits. Members of the medical establishment have repeatedly condemned its use, while those who believe in the drug have produced many reports of cures from it. Unfortunately, the evidence is more anecdotal than scientific.

Thus in 1979, when the National Cancer Institute sought to document the effectiveness of laetrile, it sent questionnaires to some 385,000 physicians and 70,000 other health professionals, and it also made direct contacts with some prolaetrile groups. Yet only ninety-three cases were submitted to the NCI for evaluation—

even though an estimated 70,000 Americans are taking laetrile. Since the sample was so small, the NCI simply concluded that nothing definite could be said about effectiveness of laetrile. The American Cancer Society also calls laetrile an "unproven method of cancer management." In June 1980 NCI announced the first clinical trial of laetrile to be carried out at four research centers for approximately 200 cancer patients. The results proved laetrile to be disappointing and ineffective.

Much of the controversy over laetrile has focused on its toxicity. In normal doses laetrile (or "vitamin B-17," as proponents call it) apparently is nontoxic. It does release cyanide, however, and larger doses can be poisonous. Backers of laetrile assert that its dangers have been exaggerated, which may be so. Still, they do exist. For example, the February 1979 issue of *The New England Journal of Medicine* reported the case of an eleven-month-old child who accidentally took one to five 500-milligram tablets. The child became ill and was taken to the hospital, where parents reported a "vitamin overdose." The child went into a coma. After taking a more detailed history, doctors determined that the "vitamin" was laetrile. Treatment for cyanide poisoning was begun, but it was too late. The baby died.

The same thing would have happened if the baby had taken an overdose of almost any potent chemotherapeutic agent. The difference, however, is that chemotherapeutic agents are given under medical supervision, while laetrile often is not.

In the long run, however, the emphasis that critics have placed on laetrile's toxicity may be misplaced. The greater danger—if the drug is truly ineffective—is that some people may be persuaded to rely on it in preference to conventional anticancer treatments that might cure them. One clinical researcher with experience at a major comprehensive cancer center said she saw no value whatever in laetrile but admitted that "as a last resort, if someone really believed in it, then I see no reason to withhold it." Another physician, a pediatrician whose medical opinions generally are on the conservative side, nevertheless maintains that cancer patients—and the parents of children with cancer—should be allowed freedom of choice up to and including the right to take laetrile.

Choice is important. Even with all of today's known cancer cures with proven response rates and proven cure rates, there are still people who will make yet another choice—to receive no modern medical treatment at all. They choose to live with the disease until they conquer it or succumb to it. For those people, laetrile, wheat grass, vitamin C, placebos, or just the power of positive thinking gives hope.

RECOMMENDED BOOKS

A *Diet Guide for Chemotherapy Patients*. 1976. 6 pp.; brochure. Ellis Fischel State Cancer Hospital, Business 70 and Garth Ave., Columbia, MO 65201. Telephone (314) 449-2711.

A *Guide to Good Nutrition During and After Chemotherapy and Radiation*, Saundra Aker, Gail Tilmont, and Vangee Harrision. 1976. 117 pp.; booklet; illus. Fred Hutchinson Cancer Research Center, Research Kitchen, 1124 Columbia St., Seattle, WA 98104. Telephone (206) 292-6301.

Blenderized Diet, Jerry Kukachka. 6 pp.; typescript. University of Wisconsin Clinical Cancer Center, Public Affairs Office, 1900 University Ave., Madison, WI 53705. Telephone (608) 262-0046.

Food for Those Who Hesitate: Tips That They Might Tolerate, Jane E. Helsel. 1976. 16 pp.; brochure. Duke University Comprehensive Cancer Center, Cancer Information Services, 200 Atlas St., Durham, NC 27705. Telephone (919) 286-2214.

Nutrition for Patients Receiving Chemotherapy and Radiation Treatment. 1974. 65 pp.; brochure. American Cancer Society, local units.

Progressive Blenderized Diet. 9 pp.; brochure. Shands Teaching Hospital and Clinics, Dept. of Food and Nutrition Services, University of Florida, Gainesville, FL 32610. Telephone (904) 392-3575.

Restricted Fiber Diet; High Protein Liquid Diet. 1968. 7 pp.; typescript. University of Wisconsin Clinical Cancer Center, Public Affairs Office, 1900 University Ave., Madison, WI 53705. Telephone (608) 262-0046.

Using Marijuana in the Reduction of Nausea Associated with Chemotherapy, Roger A. Rothman. Murray Publishing Company Inc., 2312 Third Avenue, Seattle, WA 98121. Telephone (206) 682-3560.

Chapter Twelve

The Holistic Approach

When Yvette's mother first learned that she had cancer, Yvette and her brothers found her "the best surgeon in Manhattan." Someone at the hospital mentioned visualization workshops, but Yvette ignored the suggestion. "I have always believed in the powers of the mind, but the idea that you might be able to cure cancer by visualizing healthy cells overcoming diseased ones sounded too gimmicky to me," she said.

"Then we learned mother's condition was terminal. Her physician may have been technically expert in treating cancer, but he was unfeeling. I tried to rationalize his aloof manner. I reminded myself that he treated terminal cases half the time. So how much could I expect of him? Well, when it's your own mother, believe me, what you expect is love, warmth, and understanding!"

It was at this point that Yvette's family turned to visualization. "I would have had her try anything then," said Yvette. "We also called some of the healing-prayer groups we had heard about. We are not a particularly religious family, but what has happened to my mother is what some people call a miracle."

A full year later, the prognosis for Yvette's mother remained the same: Her condition was still terminal. But she was like a new woman. Although she continued to see her physician regularly, she was not taking drugs or other treatments.

"Mother is wonderfully well, nonetheless," said Yvette. "She greets each new day with gratitude. Each new day is for her a gift of life. She enjoys this gift and lives her life to the fullest. She makes it so pleasant for everyone around her. She is a joy to be with."

The miracle that took place with Yvette's mother was not physical, but emotional. It came about as a result of a visualization workshop patterned after those conducted by a Texas couple, Dr. O. Carl Simonton and his wife, Stephanie Matthews-Simonton. Nor is it an isolated case: The same kind of change takes place in 18 to 20 percent of those cancer patients who make use of visualization therapy.

Visualization is just one of several techniques now being explored that seek to integrate the intellect, the emotions, and the body in a holistic approach to the treatment of cancer. These techniques are not really new. Prayer is one of them; another is the establishment of hospice programs for the terminally ill, inspired by the medieval hospices for travelers. What is new is that many physicians, after focusing for a long time on the body alone, are beginning to pay more attention to the ways in which health is influenced by mental and emotional state. In a sense they are returning to the rule of the father of medicine himself, Hippocrates, who is reported to have once said, "I would rather know what sort of person has the disease than what sort of disease the person has."

VISUALIZATION

The popularity of visualization therapy dates to 1976 when Dr. Simonton, a radiation oncologist, coauthored *Getting Well Again: A Step by Step Guide to Overcoming Cancer.* In this book he compares the "confused" cancer cell with the millions of other healthy cells in the body. He argues that patients can help themselves back to health by trying to "see" the healthy cells as they work to overcome the cancerous ones. He believes that "everyone participates in his or her own health or illness at all times" and that understanding how much you can participate is a significant first step for everyone in getting well.

Visualization is more than just a concept of mind over matter, or of "wishing" one's body to be well. Rather, visualization is used in conjunction with conventional medical treatments. The methods of various groups differ in details, but in addition to visualizing the healthy cells overcoming the diseased ones, the process generally includes the following steps:

• Changing one's lifestyle either to eliminate stressful situations or to compensate for a stressful job by cutting back on other activities.

• Facing one's self.

• Forgiving old hurts so completely that one can see the part one played in causing antagonism in others.

• Wishing good things—"blessings"—for those whom one dislikes.

• Maintaining a positive attitude at all times and refusing to allow negative news or feelings to interfere with one's return to health.

Confirming the value of the Simontons' approach is the experience of psychologist Neil Fiore, who reported in the February 8, 1979, *New England Journal of Medicine* on the dramatic role played by visualization therapy in his own case. After cancer of the testes metastasized to his lungs when he was just thirty-three years of age, Dr. Fiore conferred with his doctors, fully discussed and worked out the requirements for his chemotherapy, and used the holistic techniques of the Simontons. Calling upon physicians to begin fighting cancer not just with surgery and drugs, he maintained that "effective cancer therapy must treat the healthy portion of the patient's body and psyche as well as combat the diseased cells." Commenting editorially on Dr. Fiore's article, the *Journal*, often referred to as "the physician's bible," noted: "Who can quarrel with those insights? Doesn't every experienced physician know that he must deal with patients and not just their diseases? . . . If these are the lessons of holistic health, they should be welcomed as old friends. They may need fresh introduction into some of our more technologic and narrowly focused colleagues, but they nevertheless are part of the tradition of medicine."

Visualization therapy also has been espoused by Dr. Bernard S. Siegel, assistant professor of surgery at the Yale University School of Medicine, who has founded an organization called ECaPs (for *e*xceptional *ca*ncer *p*atients). He believes that only about 20 percent of all cancer patients really want to make the effort to become well. Some people, he says, "want to die, and the rest want to leave the job of recovery up to their physicians."

Dr. Siegel's figure of 20 percent who strive toward health is consistent with the Simontons'. Dr. Siegel also found an interesting parallel to those who want to live to be 100. "Whenever I speak I ask the audience how many people would like to live to be 100. Only about fifteen or twenty raise their hands." The others later explain that "they would rather die at sixty, while healthy, than lose control over their lives and be sick and linger. I think we can all learn to be healthy and live to be 100, but it does mean a change in our lifestyle. We must learn to live less stressful lives."

For many people, the hardest part of eliminating stress is forgiving others. The Simontons consider the ability to overcome resentment and to forgive so important that they devote a full chapter to it in their book. They point out that when we recognize the part we have played in creating a stressful situation and see it from the other person's point of view, it usually becomes easier to forgive and to forget.

"Religious leaders of all persuasions and philosophers of every school plead the case for forgiveness," the Simontons point out.

"They wouldn't do so if forgiving were easy. But they also would not suggest it if it were impossible."

For the cancer patient forgiveness—and the easing of the stress that it brings—can bring vast rewards. Concetta, who had been "on the outs" with a relative for many years, told how she went about it.

"It really was always like a sore spot in my heart," she said. "When I developed breast cancer and thought I didn't have very long to live, someone told me about the forgiveness idea. I realized that I at least owed it to myself to begin to feel at peace with everyone.

"But then there was that sister-in-law of mine. She had done so much to hurt me that I just couldn't see how I could forgive her. Each night I asked God to build a tiny room in my heart for her. Each day I asked that the room for her grow bigger and bigger.

"Finally I began wishing blessings for this woman. I began to realize how many things in life she needed, and I actually enjoyed wishing for her. In my mind's eye, I saw her receiving the money I knew she wanted and never had—my brother was an alcoholic who drank away most of it—and pretty soon that room for her in my heart just grew.

"One day I saw her on the street and I really couldn't muster up that old resentment anymore. I went over to her and asked how everything was, and it was just as if nothing ever happened between us."

Does visualization always work? Many people say yes. After an appearance on "The Phil Donohue Show," Dr. Siegel began receiving letters from persons across the nation who tried the techniques of visualization, participation in their treatment, and positive thinking. One woman wrote: "I was told that I had cancer nearly two years ago, and at the time, I was pregnant. I underwent breast surgery but would undergo no follow-up treatment in terms of radiation or chemotherapy though it was strongly advised. I have a healthy baby today. And I am fine. And no one knows that one of the things that helped me become well came from within me.

"Each day I began talking to my body, telling the cancer cells to behave themselves, telling my good cells to get to work, telling my body that I loved and respected it and loved the life that was within me. I began taking better care of myself, and it worked. No one even told me about it, the techniques, that is. And now I am hearing about people all across the country, and it is working for them, too."

PRAYER

Picturing the body as well, whole, and healed, despite an illness, is actually a kind of prayer written about in the 1940s by Agnes Sanford in a book called *The Healing Light*. Many religious leaders today credit Mrs. Sanford with being one of the forerunners of the visualization techniques used in the healing-through-prayer groups that have been springing up across the nation. Mrs. Sanford believes that any willing person can be used as a channel for God's healing.

During the 1960s many healing-through-prayer groups emerged in America, and gained prominence through the work of Ruth Carter Stapleton. Later, Pat Robertson's 700 Club became nationally televised through the Christian Broadcasting Network where guests often recounted stories of both physical and emotional healings. In healing-through-prayer groups, members often exhibit a very basic, realistic approach. "When we talk of miracles," said one group member, "we mean the miracles that we ourselves can bring about in our own lives . . . the miracle of living without anxiety. We have seen miracles, however, that were truly dramatic." On January 11, 1983, *Woman's Day*'s "Medical Update" section featured religious healings in Episcopalian and Roman Catholic circles.

Some groups do practice healing by the biblical technique of "laying on of hands." Some medical professionals are even doing this as part of the holistic approach to treating disease. For example, New York University professor and nurse Dolores Krieger has coined the term "therapeutic touch" for an act of healing that she teaches to other nurses. She believes that through the "therapeutic touch" she is able to transmit her own optimal energy level to the sick person, whose energy level is at a low point.

Success in visualization therapy or prayer depends largely upon the person's own involvement and willingness to believe. Regarding the matter of belief, Dr. Albert Schweitzer once noted that even a witch doctor's success was due in part to patient's expectations. "The witch doctor succeeds for the same reason all the rest of us succeed; each patient carries his own doctor inside of him. They come to us not knowing that truth. We are at our best when we give the doctor who resides within each patient a chance to go to work."

In dealing with prayer groups or visualization workshops, it is important to assess your expectations and understand the limits as well as the possibilities of such groups. One woman went into a serious depression when, despite visualization, her niece died.

"The doctors were from a big university, specialists," said Lenore. "I took my niece Juliana there. They taught her to talk to her own cancer cells, to see the good cells combating the bad ones. And we believed in it.

"But today Juliana is dead. And I feel so guilty. I told her she would live. I gave her that hope. I talked her into believing in that group, and now she is dead. I feel so guilty, so very, very guilty. Why? All that prayer. All that hope. Why?"

While Lenore saw her niece's death as a failure, those involved in prayer groups often view death as the ultimate healing. Thus prayer benefits the survivors as well as the person who is comforted by the presence of prayerful friends. For example, those in a small group in Rye, New York, who prayed for the wife of Rev. Joseph Bishop found a great peace in the experience. One woman, Gerissa, who was new to the prayer group movement, said she felt strange when asked on her first visit to pray for the minister's wife.

"I never really knew Carola," she said. "I just knew that the prayer group leader said we should spend the next twenty-four hours praying for her. Each person was to take one hour. I had heard that it began as breast cancer, but that now it had spread throughout her body. . . . Apparently there was no hope.

"My turn to pray was four in the morning, feeding time for my baby. I can still remember sitting there, the moonlight streaming through my window, shining on my child. I put the infant to my own breast and I thought of Carola. My baby was so full of life, so beautiful.

"Suddenly I found myself saying over and over again, 'Carola, you don't know me. But in the quiet of this night, I pray that somehow you can hear me. I pray for you the warmth I feel at this moment. I pray for you the joy I feel with this child. I ask that God's healing light radiate through you now, Carola, to give you new life, new health. I ask that God give you some joy, some laughter this day. Amen.'"

Carola Bishop lived two years beyond the expectation of her physicians. They were so startled that they wrote to her husband, saying, "If anything at all sustained her, it was something far beyond normal medical means." The letter was reprinted in Dr. Bishop's own book, *The Eye of the Storm*. Rev. Bishop, an early disciple of Mrs. Sanford's, has long been involved in healing through prayer groups. His theory about the healing prayer group is, "It is a phenomenon whose time has come. When there is no hope left through normal medical means, people must know that hope still exists."

THE HOSPICE MOVEMENT

When Lydia was found to have a rare and usually fatal ovarian cancer, no one ever mentioned that she might die—not her husband, not her mother, not her sister. It was a charade, a conspiracy of silence. Even her friends involved themselves in it. No one even knew who suggested it. Lydia's husband simply implied that the subject was not to be discussed.

When her sister went to visit one day, she took Carol, Lydia's closest friend, with her. "Remember," counseled Lydia's sister, "focus on her hands. They are still strong. They are still beautiful. Please try not to look surprised when you see what the chemo [chemotherapy] has done to her. And whatever you do, please don't cry."

Carol walked into the room and obliged as best she could. Lydia lifted herself up from the bed, reached out for Carol, and kissed her. As if she were ready to emerge from the curtain of secrecy that had been drawn around her in the hospital bed, Lydia said to Carol, "Pray with me. I am not afraid." The words were her last. Within moments Lydia fell into a deep sleep from which she never awakened. She never had a moment to talk about her death with her four children, her family, even her best friend.

It doesn't have to be this way.

Sarah was only thirty-three when she learned that her breast cancer had metastasized. Although she had two young children, ages two and five, Sarah turned her bedroom into a tomb the minute she heard her condition was "fatal." However, a neighbor persuaded Sarah to get in touch with the hospice team at a local hospital. The team was comprised of physicians, nurses, and other medical professionals whose primary object was to care for patients—and their families—when they are close to death.

Sarah tried to cooperate, despite the severity of her condition.

However, members of the hospice team came to her home regularly and helped her spend at least one hour a day playing with her children. In six months, when Sarah was clearly about to die, her husband was able to face this event and to talk about it with friends and, most importantly, with their children.

On Sarah's thirty-fourth birthday the team of research scientists from Sarah's laboratory—she was a biophysicist—sent her thirty-five roses. "I feel happy enough today to want to die with this much beauty around me," she said. The hospice team came to Sarah's home, dressed her children in party clothes for their mother's birthday party, and then helped Sarah play a few games with them. The next day, Sarah died.

When neighbors took the children to a Christmas party the following week, one little boy asked Sarah and Bill's children, "Are you sad that it is Christmas and you have no mommy?"

"No, we're not sad," was the reply. "She was very sick, but she played with us every day. We miss her. But we are happy that she won't ever be sick again."

The primary difference in the deaths of Lydia and Sarah was the effect that they had on the children. Lydia's four children, aged six, eight, ten, and fourteen, were shocked that their mother had died. They were depressed and had difficulty coping. Sarah's children, despite their ages, seemed to adjust to life without their mother. Her husband attributes this to the hospice team.

Throughout the world hospice centers are opening for terminal patients of all ages. While many people think of hospice as a place to die, in concept it is a place to live. Many centers offer creative workshops. The term *hospice* goes back to the middle ages, when hospices were way stations, often set up by monks or nuns for weary travelers. The most famous ones were those of the Great and Little St. Bernard Passes in the Alps. The modern kind of hospice dates to the mid-1960s, when Dr. Cicely Saunders established St. Christopher's Hospice in London to provide care for the dying. Patterned after St. Christopher's Hospice, some seventy-five to one hundred centers are in operation—or about to begin operation—in the United States today.

The popularity of the hospice concept is partly a reflection of the high cost of medical technology, especially in cases of intensive care, including the care of the terminally ill. It is simply cheaper to stay in a modest hotel-like facility than in a large hospital with all the expensive trappings of modern medicine. The popularity of hospices also is due in part to the common perception of hospitals as cold, unfeeling institutions. However, the hospice concept also differs from traditional ideas of health care in at least four basic ways:

• The patient together with his or her family is considered the unit of care, not just the patient alone.

• An interdisciplinary team is used to assess the physical, psychological, and spiritual needs of the patient and the family, and to develop and provide an overall, coordinated plan of care.

• Pain and the collateral symptoms associated with terminal illness and its previous treatment are controlled, but no heroic efforts are made to cure the patient.

• The hospice team does not cease its efforts at death but continues to help the family to overcome emotional suffering afterward.

Some patients may choose to go to a hospice center, while others will prefer to remain at home and die in their own beds—the normal procedure for many of our grandparents and great-grandparents. It is only within the last generation or so that people have started to go to a hospital to die. For women with children, such as Sarah, staying at home often is preferable. In either case, though, the objective of the hospice program is still to involve the family whenever possible in helping the woman, or man, to accept death as a natural part of human existence.

What many persons have found most valuable about the hospice program is the bereavement counseling offered by the hospice team members after a person's death. "Bereavement counseling is a crucial part of helping family members adjust to living after the death of someone whom they love."

The emotional support that the dying person receives from the hospice staff also is most important. Dying patients in hospitals without hospice units frequently have to deal with physicians and other staff members who themselves are deeply troubled by the idea of death and adopt different methods of evading it.

Some physicians and nurses can hardly bear to face a patient who is approaching death. In fact the "runner," the "snowman," and the "biochemist" are well-known characters in hospital life. The first is the doctor or nurse who pops into a room, says, "Hello, how are you?" and pops out of the room before an answer can be given. The snowman, meanwhile, greets the dying patient with glacial coolness. No genuine emotion comes through, even when the snowman adopts an air of conviviality: it is forced. As for the biochemist, this is the staff member who pays close attention to the technical details of fluids, drug dosage, temperature, and calories consumed but rarely looks into the eyes of the patient or speaks of anything with any real emotion. Naturally, most patients sense these rejections and withdraw, looking no more to the emotionally frozen professionals for help.

The runner, the snowman, and the biochemist are common but not typical. Most professionals are warm and loving, and they extend themselves in many ways to give support to the patient with a terminal disease. Although it is a difficult thing to prove scientifically, most physicians and nurses believe that the patient who is surrounded by supportive and compassionate professionals will respond better to treatment. In fact many hospitals—influenced to some extent by the hospice concept—are developing their own liaison psychiatry teams to work with the terminally ill, as well as with their families, their friends, and, last but by no means least, the physicians who treat them.

At the same time, not all physicians are in favor of the hospice concept, at least not in the form of centers that are separate from conventional hospitals. In a society that clearly does not have unlimited funds to support health care, they see dangers in creating an alternate terminal-care system. Today no one goes to a hospice unless he or she wants to, but is it possible that some day people might be assigned to terminal-care facilities? "Who makes the decision for hospice and when is it made?" asks one doctor. "Just the existence of this terminal facility presupposes the possibility of making errors in determination and sending some people to their end prematurely. And if an error is to be made, isn't it better to prolong life too often rather than to shorten it even once?"

Nor is a hospice center the right answer for every patient. Many women feel that to go into a center is to give up, to lose all hope, and this is something they cannot bear. To them this is synonymous with death itself. They would rather keep on fighting, no matter what the pain and the cost, even if their only hope is a miracle. By continuing treatment—and sometimes by accepting frankly experimental or "heroic" treatments—they may prolong their lives. If they are fortunate, they may live comfortably and usefully. If nothing else, what they do may contribute to the war against cancer. The experience physicians gain with new treatment plans may lead to help for future patients.

Such heroics bought time for Nancy Jane, who lived eight years beyond the expectations of her physicians. Nancy Jane was afraid to die and wouldn't hear of it at twenty. She filled her life with planning minute details of parties and working at jobs that allowed her to continue new treatments. "I'm a guinea pig. I know it. And I don't care. But I refuse to let this horrible disease be for nothing."

When she was twenty-eight, Nancy Jane decided she had had

enough. Yet once in the hospital and faced with death, she asked her doctors to find still another experimental technique. Finally the doctors said, "Your body just won't take any more. We're sorry."

Nancy Jane went home angry and furious for a few days. Then she decided to plan her send-off. Her two best friends from school joined her as she wrote her obituary and planned "her" party—an outdoor garden party—to be held after the funeral. Then followed one week of great difficulty. Nancy Jane drifted in and out of coma. Her family and friends spent another full week with her around the clock. Then her best friend, Jean, said, "Nancy Jane, we've watched you suffer long enough. We've watched you live and we're going to stay with you until you die. So please say goodbye to all of us now, close your eyes, and while we hold your hand start looking for someone to help you cross over into your next life.

"We won't leave you till someone comes for you. Watch for someone. Take their hand. Then go, Nancy Jane. We're going to miss you. We won't ever forget you . . . you've made our lives so special, because you were so special. Goodbye, Nancy Jane."

Within moments, Nancy Jane smiled, let go of her friends' hands, and waved goodbye.

Nancy Jane had striven for the impossible, but the effort was worthwhile for her—and perhaps for others.

The gains made in the treatment of children with cancer may well have come about because their mothers begged for the impossible. In *Conquering Cancer*, Dr. Lucien Israel says, "It is easy to say to the relatives of an adult, 'Let's bow to the inevitable, there is nothing to be done.' It was not so easy to say that to the mothers of young children with leukemia, who begged doctors to attempt the impossible and take risks. This is one reason—and there are many others—why advances were made more rapidly in childhood leukemia than in other tumors. The hematologists really did attempt the impossible."

THE RIGHT TO CHOOSE

Implicit in the hospice concept is the right to know that one's condition is terminal. If the patient does not know, then it is impossible to choose between hospice and hospital, between dying at home and undergoing all the "heroic" treatments that modern medicine has to offer. The individual should have the right to make an informed choice.

Olivia, for example, was a deeply compassionate woman who lived what she said was a "good life." Life had been kind to Olivia, her husband, and her children. She never even recalled being seriously ill.

One day Olivia could not get out of bed. She had her son call the physician and then asked to see her sisters who lived on the same block. The family gathered at Olivia's home within minutes, and then she told them the story that stunned them all.

"Last year, I learned that I had cancer. Because I could not in any way consider surgery or treatments, I asked the doctor to just let me go quietly about my business. I was assured that when the time came, I would be given medicine to keep me comfortable, and you would all be given a great deal of supportive help.

"I don't wish to go into a hospice center. I want to stay here with all of you whom I have loved so much. This was my choice then. It is my choice now. Please support me."

Did Olivia's physician err in allowing her life to be shortened? No. She was told of all her options and she made her own choice. She didn't want a hospice or a hospital. She didn't particularly want to talk about death, either. She didn't want "heroics." She just wanted home.

Other women will make other choices.

To Alicia, who was told her cancer was terminal twenty-five years ago and tried everything, heroics were worth it.

To Genevieve, who tried everything from chemotherapy to hyperthermia to visualization therapy to wheat grass before she went on laetrile and then back onto a new chemotherapeutic drug, heroics were worth it. After all, she lived to see her daughter married and her first grandchild born. And that was all she said she ever wanted to live to see. It meant staying alive for twelve years to see it. "Heroics," said Genevieve, "hell, yes."

To mothers who have seen their children with cancer and who have pleaded with doctors to "do everything" when the child lived, the heroics were worth it.

But how can women make these decisions if they are not told the nature of their disease? And most people, it seems, do want to be told. In a 1979 Gallup survey, Drs. Norman B. Levy and Michael Blumenfield asked more than 1,000 people the question, "If you had a terminal illness, would you want to be told about it or not?" Nine of ten people responded yes, with relatively more men than women answering this way. Some physicians interpreted the discrepancy to mean that fewer women needed to be told outright. They felt that some women "instinctively" know—which may or may not be true. What is certain is that the physician does not always have to announce to a woman that she has cancer. Patients are aware of their physical condition and they pick up many nonvocal clues from their physicians.

Nonetheless, the problem of telling or not telling remains a very real one, even for those with much experience in caring for patients with terminal disease. Many well-meaning families actually will say to the physician, "*Don't* tell her she has cancer." If the physician complies, he or she becomes an accomplice in the plot against the patient. Sooner or later, the woman will discover she has cancer, and then she will be prevented from having frank discussion with her physician. She will feel that the family is trying to hide the truth, and she will lose much of the support they offer as well. Fabricating the truth tends to create more pain and alienation for dying patients.

On the other hand, it is not necessary for a woman with terminal cancer to be constantly beaten down with the nature of her disease. The preferred course is honesty. But honesty may mean honest emotions and honest intent, rather than a complete explanation of every technical detail of the dying patient's metabolism.

Drs. Levy and Blumenfield undertook a second survey, this time at Downstate Medical Center, to determine whether physicians would in fact tell dying patients the truth. Ninety percent of the physicians, residents, and students at Downstate Medical Center in Brooklyn, New York, said yes, they would inform a patient.

Despite this result, Levy and Blumenfield themselves did not believe there should be a fixed approach to telling or not telling. "Patients should not have the information forced upon them," they said, while urging that "those who deal with the terminally ill . . . understand their needs and wishes and make a decision that is really in the patient's best interest." However, they concluded that "if we as psychiatrists were asked the question, 'Should a patient be told of a fatal illness'? we would have to answer, 'I don't know.'"

As an example of a person who did not really want to be told, Dr. Levy related the story of his first wife, who was in her early thirties when it was discovered that she had breast cancer. "With three young children under the age of six, it was important for her to feel that she would live. Not only did she want to believe that she would live, she never wanted any discussion of death. I understood her need and so would go so far as to call physicians and technicians when she was going back to the hospital for treatment to make certain that they never at any time mentioned the fact that her case was terminal.

"When she went to the hospital for the last time, we didn't discuss death, but she knew. 'This will be my last trip there,' she said."

Frequently, the dying patient will make it clear—as did Dr. Levy's wife—in what manner he or she wishes to be treated. This may or may not be done explicitly with instructions such as, "I want to talk about this," or "I don't want to talk about that." There are many kinds of clues that the sensitive, compassionate physician, friend, or family member will pick up concerning the appropriate path to follow. No generalizations are safe and no generalizations are useful.

Some dying women will be consumed by grief and frustration; others will rush to complete unfinished business. Some may quietly review the past and await the inevitable; some may madly charge about displaying anger; some may look for false promises to support their flagging hopes. How a woman deals with her fate is deeply personal. What is crucial is the support that she and her family receive.

Some women actually manage to dismiss the idea that they have cancer. They develop what is known as "the block." After going through the fear, pain, and anguish of the diagnosis, they mask their thoughts and emotions so completely that they themselves are not aware of them. This does not always prevent them from cooperating in their own treatment.

If all physicians were to routinely prepare patients for visits from persons trained to help women deal with the emotional aspects of the cancer, more women would benefit. Unfortunately, because so many physicians feel that *they* know best about handling their patients, they sometimes resent the efforts of psychiatric teams or volunteer groups.

Dr. Alfred M. Freedman, Chairman of the Department of Psychiatry and Behaviorial Sciences at New York Medical College, says that one of the most common complaints heard from women who have had cancer is the lack of empathy and understanding on the part of the treating physician. "Not all physicians deal with patients on an impersonal level," he says, "but many do not encourage women to express their deepest feelings, fears and concerns about their illness.

"Women often say that when they ultimately are told they have cancer, it is catastrophic, and it takes all of their inner resources and reasoning to keep them from panicking. For many women, it is not just the cancer that they must deal with, but the daily events of life, a family, or children, or a job, perhaps. Often they go into surgery feeling burdened and incapable of coping.

"Helping women to adjust, to cope, is important. I do not feel that every woman needs to be treated by a psychiatrist, but I do feel that they should be treated by physicians who give them a sense of personal worth, a sense of importance. Many women can still lead productive lives despite the disease. Women must be made to feel valuable, not just because they are women, but because they are individuals. Women with cancer—just as all women and men—have needs and wants that must be met. Women with cancer, however, often have special needs that must be respected and met with a special sense of caring."

No matter how well adjusted a woman you might be, do not be discouraged by your own feelings if you become fearful or depressed. Nor should you consider yourself "strange" if you can maintain an exceedingly positive attitude. You need not apologize for your emotions. You feel what you feel. If you sense the need for an understanding trained professional, do ask to see a liaison psychiatrist. Some hospitals provide such help on a routine basis.

Do contact the American Cancer Society for a list of support groups in your area to help you and your family adjust to living with cancer. New ones are being formed every day. In support groups, you will find that you are not alone in your fears, your feelings, and your desire for warmth and understanding.

Appendix A

COMPREHENSIVE CANCER CENTERS

Below is a list of the major cancer centers in the United States.

Alabama
Comprehensive Cancer Center
University of Alabama in Birmingham
University Station
Birmingham, Alabama 35294
Phone: (205) 934-5077

California
Los Angeles County-University of Southern California Comprehensive Cancer Center
2025 Zonal Avenue
Los Angeles, California 90033
Phone: (213) 226-2008

UCLA Comprehensive Cancer Center
UCLA School of Medicine
924 Westwood Boulevard, Suite 650
Los Angeles, California 90024
Phone: (213) 825-2532
(213) 825-5268

Colorado
Colorado Regional Cancer Center, Inc.
165 Cook Street
Denver, Colorado 80206
Phone: (303) 320-5921

Connecticut
Yale University Comprehensive Cancer Center
333 Cedar Street
New Haven, Connecticut 06510
Phone: (203) 432-4122

District of Columbia
Georgetown University/Howard University
Comprehensive Cancer Center
Vincent T. Lombardi Cancer Research Center
Georgetown University Medical Center
3800 Reservoir Road, N.W.
Washington, D.C. 20007
Phone: (202) 625-7066

Howard University Cancer Research Center
College of Medicine
Washington, D.C. 20059
Phone: (202) 745-1406

Florida
Comprehensive Cancer Center for the State of Florida
University of Miami School of Medicine/Jackson Memorial Medical Center
P.O. Box 520875, Biscayne Annex
Miami, Florida 33134
Phone: (305) 545-6758

Illinois
Illinois Cancer Council
37 S. Wabash Avenue
Chicago, Illinois 60603
Phone: (312) 346-9813

Maryland
Johns Hopkins Oncology Center
601 North Broadway
Baltimore, Maryland 21205
Phone: (301) 955-8822

Massachusetts
Sidney Farber Cancer Institute
44 Binney Street
Boston, Massachusetts 02115
Phone: (617) 732-3555

Michigan
Cancer Center of Metropolitan Detroit
110 East Warren Avenue
Detroit, Michigan 48201
Phone: (313) 833-0710

Minnesota
Mayo Comprehensive Cancer Center
200 First Street, S.W.
Rochester, Minnesota 55901
Phone: (507) 282-2511

New York
Memorial Sloan-Kettering Cancer Center
1275 York Avenue
New York, New York 10021
Phone: (212) 794-7585

Roswell Park Memorial Institute
666 Elm Street
Buffalo, New York 14263
Phone: (716) 845-5770

North Carolina
Comprehensive Cancer Center
Duke University Medical Center
P.O. Box 3814
Durham, North Carolina 27710
Phone: (919) 684-2282

Ohio
Ohio State University Comprehensive Cancer Center
357 McCampbell Drive
Columbus, Ohio 43210
Phone: (614) 422-5022

Pennsylvania
Fox Chase/University of Pennsylvania Comprehensive Cancer Center
The Fox Chase Cancer Center
7701 Burholme Avenue
Philadelphia, Pennsylvania 19111
Phone: (215) 342-1000

University of Pennsylvania Cancer Center
578 Maloney Building
3400 Spruce Street
Philadelphia, Pennsylvania 19104
Phone: (215) 662-3910

Texas
The University of Texas System-Cancer Center
M.D. Anderson Hospital and Tumor Institute
6723 Bertner Avenue
Houston, Texas 77030
Phone: (713) 792-3000

Washington
Fred Hutchinson Cancer Research Center
1124 Columbia Street
Seattle, Washington 98104
Phone: (206) 292-2930

Wisconsin
The University of Wisconsin Clinical Cancer Center
1300 University Avenue
Madison, Wisconsin 53706
Phone: (608) 263-2553

Appendix B

APPROVED CANCER PROGRAMS

Criteria for Categorization

Only cancer programs approved by the American College of Surgeons are published here. *See pages 20–21 for a discussion of the six categories of approved programs.*

Support

The American College of Surgeons conducts this project under grant and contract support from the American Cancer Society, Inc., and the National Cancer Institute, Department of Health, Education, and Welfare.

Additional Information

Reprints of this list are mailed without charge to each institution named and to agencies in the field of cancer control.

Orders for the *Cancer Program Manual*, additional copies of this list, and other informational literature, as well as all inquiries concerning the up-to-date status of an institution's cancer program, should be addressed to: *The Commission on Cancer, American College of Surgeons, 55 East Erie Street, Chicago, Illinois 60611.*

Alabama

Birmingham

University of Alabama Hospitals
Veterans Administration Medical Center

Mobile

University of South Alabama Medical Center—Hospitals and Clinics

Tuskegee

Veterans Administration Medical Center

Alaska

Anchorage

Alaska Hospital and Medical Center
USPHS Alaska Native Medical Center

Fairbanks

Fairbanks Memorial Hospital

Arizona

Flagstaff

Flagstaff Hospital and Medical Center of Northern Arizona

Mesa

Desert Samaritan Hospital and Health Center
Mesa Lutheran Hospital

Phoenix

Good Samaritan Hospital
Maricopa County General Hospital
Memorial Hospital
Veterans Administration Medical Center

Scottsdale

Scottsdale Memorial Hospital

Tucson

Tucson Medical Center
University Hospital
Veterans Administration Medical Center

Arkansas

Fayetteville

Washington Regional Medical Center

Fort Smith

Sparks Regional Medical Center

Little Rock

University Hospital
Veterans Administration Medical Center

Texarkana

St. Michael Hospital

California

Alhambra

Alhambra Community Hospital

Anaheim

Anaheim Memorial Hospital
Martin Luther Hospital Medical Center

Arcadia

Methodist Hospital of Southern California

Bakersfield

Kern Medical Center
San Joaquin Community Hospital

Bellflower

Bellwood General Hospital
Kaiser Foundation Hospital

Berkeley

Alta Bates Hospital
Herrick Hospital and Health Center

Burbank
St. Joseph Medical Center
Canoga Park
West Hills Medical Center
Chico
N. T. Enloe Memorial Hospital
Concord
Mount Diablo Hospital Medical Center
Covina
Inter-Community Hospital
Culver City
Brotman Medical Center
Duarte
City of Hope National Medical Center
Santa Teresita Hospital
Fontana
Kaiser Foundation Hospital
Fountain Valley
Fountain Valley Community Hospital
Fresno
Fresno Community Hospital and Medical Center
Valley Children's Hospital
Veterans Administration Medical Center
Glendale
Glendale Adventist Medical Center
Glendale Community Hospital
Memorial Hospital of Glendale
Granada Hills
Granada Hills Community Hospital
Harbor City
Kaiser Foundation Hospital
Imola
Napa State Hospital
Inglewood
Centinela Hospital Medical Center
Daniel Freeman Memorial Hospital
Laguna Hills
Southern Orange County Cancer Program
Saddleback Community Hospital, *Laguna Hills*
Mission Community Hospital, *Mission Viejo*
San Clemente General Hospital, *San Clemente*
South Coast Community Hospital, *South Laguna*
La Jolla
Green Hospital of Scripps Clinic
Scripps Memorial Hospital
La Mesa
Grossmont District Hospital
Livermore
Veterans Administration Medical Center
Loma Linda
Loma Linda University Medical Center
Long Beach
Long Beach Community Hospital
Los Altos Hospital
Memorial Hospital Medical Center of Long Beach
Naval Regional Medical Center
St. Mary Medical Center—Bauer Hospital
Veterans Administration Medical Center
Los Angeles
California Hospital Medical Center
Childrens Hospital of Los Angeles

Hollywood Presbyterian Medical Center
Hospital of the Good Samaritan
Kaiser Foundation Hospital—Cadillac
Kaiser Foundation Hospital—Sunset
Los Angeles County, USC Medical Center
Martin Luther King, Jr. General Hospital
Orthopaedic Hospital Medical Center
Queen of Angels Hospital
St. Vincent Medical Center
UCLA Hospital
White Memorial Medical Center

Lynwood
St. Francis Medical Center

Martinez
Veterans Administration Medical Center

Modesto
Memorial Hospitals Association

Montebello
Beverly Hospital

Monterey Park
Garfield Medical Center

Newport Beach
Hoag Memorial Hospital Presbyterian

Northridge
Northridge Hospital Foundation

Oakland
Naval Regional Medical Center
Samuel Merritt Hospital

Oceanside
Tri-City Hospital

Orange
St. Joseph Hospital
University of California Irvine Medical Center

Oxnard
St. John's Hospital

Palm Springs
Desert Hospital

Panorama City
Kaiser Foundation Hospital

Pasadena
Huntington Memorial Hospital
St. Luke Hospital of Pasadena

Pomona
Pomona Valley Community Hospital

Rancho Mirage
Eisenhower Medical Center

Redlands
Redlands Community Hospital

Redondo Beach
South Bay Hospital

Redwood City
Sequoia Hospital District

Riverside
Parkview Community Hospital
Riverside Community Hospital
Riverside General Hospital—University Medical Center

Sacramento
Mercy General Hospital
Sutter Community Hospitals of Sacramento
University of California—Davis Medical Center

San Bernardino
St. Bernadine Hospital
San Bernardino Community Hospital

San Bernardino (cont.)
San Bernardino County Medical Center

San Diego
Children's Hospital & Health Center
Donald N. Sharp Memorial Community Hospital
Kaiser Foundation Hospital
Mercy Hospital and Medical Center
Naval Regional Medical Center
University Hospital

San Dimas
Combined Hospital Cancer Program
Foothill Presbyterian Hospital, *Glendora*
Glendora Community Hospital, *Glendora*
San Dimas Community Hospital, *San Dimas*
West Covina Hospital, *West Covina*

San Francisco
Children's Hospital of San Francisco
French Hospital/Medical Center
Letterman Army Medical Center
Mount Zion Hospital and Medical Center
Ralph K. Davies Medical Center—Franklin Hospital
St. Francis Memorial Hospital
St. Mary's Hospital and Medical Center
San Francisco General Hospital Medical Center
USPHS Hospital
University of California Hospitals and Clinics
Veterans Administration Medical Center

San Gabriel
Community Hospital of San Gabriel

San Jose
O'Connor Hospital
San Jose Health Center
Santa Clara Valley Medical Center

San Pablo
Brookside Hospital

San Pedro
San Pedro Peninsula Hospital

Santa Ana
Santa Ana-Tustin Community Hospital

Santa Barbara
Santa Barbara Cottage Hospital

Santa Monica
St. John's Hospital and Health Center
Santa Monica Hospital Medical Center

Stockton
Dameron Hospital

Tarzana
Medical Center of Tarzana Hospital

Thousand Oaks
Los Robles Regional Medical Center

Torrance
Los Angeles County Harbor—UCLA Medical Center
Torrance Memorial Hospital Medical Center

Travis AFB
David Grant USAF Medical Center

Upland
San Antonio Community Hospital

Van Nuys
Valley Presbyterian Hospital
Visalia
Kaweah Delta District Hospital
Walnut Creek
John Muir Memorial Hospital
Whittier
Presbyterian Intercommunity Hospital

Colorado
Colorado Springs
Penrose Hospital
Denver
Fitzsimons Army Medical Center, *Aurora*
Porter/Swedish Cancer Program
Porter Memorial Hospital
Swedish Medical Center, *Englewood*
Presbyterian Medical Center
Rose Medical Center
St. Anthony Hospital Systems
Saint Joseph Hospital
St. Luke's Hospital
University of Colorado Health Sciences Center—University Hospital
Veterans Administration Medical Center
Fort Carson
US Army Hospital
Fort Collins
Poudre Valley Memorial Hospital
Greeley
Weld County General Hospital
Lakewood
AMC Cancer Research Center and Hospital
Longmont
Longmont United Hospital
Montrose
Montrose Memorial Hospital
Pueblo
St. Mary-Corwin Hospital
USAF Academy
USAF Academy Hospital
Wheat Ridge
Lutheran Medical Center

Connecticut
Bridgeport
Bridgeport Hospital
Park City Hospital
St. Vincent's Medical Center
Danbury
Danbury Hospital
Derby
Griffin Hospital
Farmington
University of Connecticut Health Center, John Dempsey Hospital
Greenwich
Greenwich Hospital Association
Groton
Naval Submarine Medical Center
Hartford
Hartford Hospital
Mount Sinai Hospital
Saint Francis Hospital and Medical Center
Meriden
Meriden-Wallingford Hospital
New Haven
Hospital of St. Raphael
Yale-New Haven Hospital
Norwalk
Norwalk Hospital

Norwich
The William W. Backus Hospital
Stamford
St. Joseph Hospital
Stamford Hospital
Torrington
Charlotte Hungerford Hospital
Waterbury
St. Mary's Hospital
Waterbury Hospital

Delaware
Lewes
Beebe Hospital of Sussex County
Wilmington
Veterans Administration Medical Center
Wilmington Medical Center

District of Columbia
Washington
Children's Hospital National Medical Center
Georgetown University Hospital
Greater Southeast Community Hospital
Howard University Hospital
Walter Reed Army Medical Center

Florida
Daytona Beach
Halifax Hospital Medical Center
Dunedin
Mease Hospital and Clinic
Gainesville
Shands Teaching Hospital and Clinics
Jacksonville
Memorial Hospital of Jacksonville
Naval Regional Medical Center
St. Vincent's Medical Center
University Hospital of Jacksonville
Miami
James M. Jackson Memorial Hospital
Pensacola
Naval Aerospace and Regional Medical Center
West Florida Hospital
Tallahassee
Tallahassee Memorial Regional Medical Center
Tampa
St. Joseph's Hospital
Tampa General Hospital

Georgia
Albany
Phoebe Putney Memorial Hospital
Americus
Americus and Sumter County Hospital
Atlanta
Crawford W. Long Memorial Hospital
Emory University Hospital
Georgia Baptist Medical Center
Grady Memorial Hospital
Piedmont Hospital
St. Joseph's Hospital
West Paces Ferry Hospital
Augusta
Eugene Talmadge Memorial Hospital—Medical College of Georgia
University Hospital
Austell
Cobb General Hospital

Columbus
Medical Center
Dalton
Hamilton Memorial Hospital
Decatur
De Kalb General Hospital
Veterans Administration Hospital Atlanta
East Point
South Fulton Hospital
Fort Benning
Martin Army Hospital
Fort Gordon
Dwight D. Eisenhower Army Medical Center
Gainesville
Northeast Georgia Medical Center
La Grange
West Georgia Medical Center/ Enoch Callaway Cancer Clinic
Macon
Medical Center of Central Georgia
Savannah
Memorial Medical Center
Tifton
Tift General Hospital
Valdosta
South Georgia Medical Center

Hawaii
Honolulu
Kaiser Foundation Hospital
Kapiolani Hospital
Kuakini Medical Center
Queen's Medical Center
St. Francis Hospital
Tripler Army Medical Center

Idaho
Boise
St. Luke's Hospital & Mountain States Tumor Institute
Lewiston
St. Joseph's Hospital
Nampa
Mercy Medical Center
Twin Falls
Magic Valley Memorial Hospital

Illinois
Arlington Heights
Northwest Community Hospital
Aurora
Copley Memorial Hospital
Berwyn
MacNeal Memorial Hospital
Carbondale
Memorial Hospital of Carbondale
Chicago
Bethesda Hospital
Central Community Hospital
Children's Memorial Hospital
Columbus Hospital
Cook County Hospital
Edgewater Hospital
Franklin Boulevard Community Hospital
Holy Cross Hospital
Illinois Masonic Medical Center
Louis A. Weiss Memorial Hospital
Mercy Hospital and Medical Center
Mount Sinai Hospital Medical Center of Chicago
Northwestern Memorial Hospital
Ravenswood Hospital Medical Center

Chicago (cont.)
Rush-Presbyterian-St. Luke's Medical Center
St. Elizabeth's Hospital
St. Joseph Hospital
Saint Mary of Nazareth Hospital Center
Swedish Covenant Hospital
University of Chicago Hospitals and Clinics
University of Illinois Hospital
Veterans Administration West Side Medical Center

Chicago Heights
St. James Hospital

Danville
Lakeview Medical Center
St. Elizabeth Hospital

Decatur
Decatur Memorial Hospital

Effingham
St. Anthony's Memorial Hospital

Elgin
Saint Joseph Hospital
Sherman Hospital

Elk Grove Village
Alexian Brothers Medical Center

Elmhurst
Memorial Hospital of DuPage County

Evanston
Evanston Hospital
St. Francis Hospital of Evanston

Evergreen Park
Little Company of Mary Hospital

Great Lakes
Naval Regional Medical Center

Harvey
Ingalls Memorial Hospital

Hinsdale
Hinsdale Sanitarium and Hospital

Kankakee
St. Mary's Hospital of Kankakee

Lake Forest
Lake Forest Hospital

Libertyville
Condell Memorial Hospital

Maywood
Foster G. McGaw Hospital

McHenry
McHenry Hospital

Moline
Lutheran Hospital

Oak Lawn
Christ Hospital

Oak Park
West Suburban Hospital

Park Ridge
Lutheran General Hospital

Peoria
Methodist Medical Center of Illinois
St. Francis Hospital Medical Center

Quincy
Blessing Hospital
St. Mary Hospital

Rockford
Rockford Memorial Hospital
St. Anthony Hospital-Medical Center
Swedish-American Hospital

Skokie
Skokie Valley Community Hospital

Sterling
Community General Hospital

Streator
St. Mary's Hospital

Urbana
Carle Foundation Hospital

Indiana
Bluffton
Caylor-Nickel Hospital
East Chicago
St. Catherine Hospital of East Chicago, Indiana, Inc.
Evansville
Deaconess Hospital
Welborn Baptist Hospital
Gary
Methodist Hospital of Gary
Hammond
St. Margaret Hospital
Indianapolis
Community Hospital of Indianapolis
Methodist Hospital of Indiana
St. Vincent Hospital and Health Care Center
Lafayette
St. Elizabeth Hospital Medical Center
Terre Haute
Terre Haute Regional Hospital
Union Hospital
Vincennes
Good Samaritan Hospital

Iowa
Des Moines
Iowa Methodist Medical Center
Mercy Hospital Medical Center
Veterans Administration Medical Center
Dubuque
Finley Hospital
Mercy Health Center—St. Joseph's Unit
Xavier Hospital
Iowa City
University of Iowa Hospitals and Clinics

Kansas
Fort Riley
Irwin Army Hospital
Hays
Hadley Regional Medical Center
St. Anthony Hospital
Kansas City
Bethany Medical Center
University of Kansas Medical Center
Manhattan
Memorial/Saint Mary Hospitals Cancer Program
Memorial Hospital
The Saint Mary Hospital
Wichita
St. Francis Hospital of Wichita, Inc.
St. Joseph Medical Center
Veterans Administration Medical and Regional Office Center
Wesley Medical Center

Kentucky
Fort Campbell
United States Army Hospital
Lexington
Good Samaritan Hospital
University Hospital
Louisville
Highlands Baptist Hospital
Norton-Children's Hospital, Inc.,

Norton Memorial Infirmary
University Hospital, Louisville General Hospital
Veterans Administration Medical Center
Madisonville
Regional Medical Center of Hopkins County

Louisiana
Alexandria
Alexandria Tumor Registry Program
Rapides General Hospital
St. Francis Cabrini Hospital
Eunice
Moose Memorial Hospital
Lake Charles
St. Patrick Hospital of Lake Charles
New Orleans
Charity Hospital of Louisiana at New Orleans
Touro Infirmary
USPHS Hospital
Veterans Administration Medical Center
Shreveport
Louisiana State University Hospital
Veterans Administration Medical Center

Maine
Augusta
Augusta General Hospital
Bangor
Eastern Maine Medical Center
Lewiston
Central Maine Medical Center
St. Mary's General Hospital
Norway
Stephens Memorial Hospital
Portland
Maine Medical Center
Presque Isle
Arthur Gould Memorial Hospital
Rockland
Penobscot Bay Medical Center
Togus
Veterans Administration Medical Center
Waterville
Mid-Maine Medical Center

Maryland
Andrews AFB
Malcolm Grow USAF Medical Center
Baltimore
Franklin Square Hospital
Greater Baltimore Medical Center
Johns Hopkins Hospital
Sinai Hospital of Baltimore
South Baltimore General Hospital
USPHS Hospital
University of Maryland Hospital
Bethesda
National Naval Medical Center
Leonardtown
St. Mary's Hospital
Salisbury
Peninsula General Hospital Medical Center
Towson
St. Joseph Hospital

Massachusetts
Beverly
Beverly Hospital

Boston
Beth Israel Hospital
Boston City Hospital
Brigham and Women's Hospital
Carney Hospital
Children's Hospital Medical Center
Faulkner Hospital, *Jamaica Plain*
Lahey Clinic Foundation
Massachusetts General Hospital
New England Deaconess Hospital
St. Elizabeth's Hospital of Boston, *Brighton*
USPHS Hospital, *Brighton*
University Hospital
Veterans Administration Medical Center, *Jamaica Plain*

Brockton
Brockton Hospital
Cardinal Cushing General Hospital

Cambridge
Mount Auburn Hospital

Chelsea
Lawrence F. Quigley Memorial Hospital Soldier's Home in Massachusetts

Concord
Emerson Hospital

Danvers
Hunt Memorial Hospital

Framingham
Framingham Union Hospital

Holyoke
Holyoke Hospital
Providence Hospital

Hyannis
Cape Cod Hospital

Lynn
Lynn Hospital

Medford
Lawrence Memorial Hospital of Medford

Newton Lower Falls
Newton-Wellesley Hospital

North Adams
North Adams Regional Hospital

Northampton
The Cooley Dickenson Hospital

Norwood
Norwood Hospital

Pittsfield
Berkshire Medical Center

Plymouth
The Jordan Hospital

Salem
Salem Hospital

Springfield
Baystate Medical Center
Mercy Hospital

Stoughton
Goddard Memorial Hospital

Walpole
Pondville Hospital

Waltham
The Waltham Hospital

Winchester
Winchester Hospital

Worcester
St. Vincent Hospital
The Memorial Hospital
Worcester City Hospital

Michigan

Allen Park
Veterans Administration Medical Center

Ann Arbor
St. Joseph Mercy Hospital
University Hospital
Battle Creek
Calhoun County Medical Society Cancer Program
Battle Creek Sanitarium Hospital
Community Hospital Association
Leila Y. Post Montgomery Hospital
Dearborn
Oakwood Hospital
Detroit
Detroit General Hospital
Harper-Grace Hospitals
Henry Ford Hospital
Flint
Hurley Medical Center
St. Joseph Hospital
Grand Rapids
Blodgett Memorial Medical Center
Butterworth Hospital
Ferguson-Droste-Ferguson Hospital
St. Mary's Hospital
Lansing
Edward W. Sparrow Hospital
Menominee
Marinette, WT-Menominee Cancer Program
Menominee County Lloyd Hospital
Muskegon
Hackley Hospital and Medical Center
Rochester
Crittenton Hospital
Royal Oak
William Beaumont Hospital
Southfield
Providence Hospital

Minnesota
Crookston
Riverview Hospital Association
Fergus Falls
Lake Region Hospital
Grand Rapids
Itasca Memorial Hospital
Hibbing
Central Mesabi Medical Center
Minneapolis
Abbott-Northwestern Hospital
Children's Health Center & Hospital
Metropolitan Medical Center
St. Mary's Hospital
University of Minnesota Hospitals and Clinics
Veterans Administration Medical Center
Moorhead
St. Ansgar Hospital
Rochester
Mayo Clinic
St. Louis Park
Methodist Hospital

Mississippi
Biloxi
Howard Memorial Hospital
Veterans Administration Medical Center
Hattiesburg
Forrest County General Hospital

Jackson
University Hospital
Veterans Administration Medical Center
Keesler AFB
USAF Medical Center
Pascagoula
Singing River Hospital
Vicksburg
Mercy Regional Medical Center

Missouri
Cape Girardeau
St. Francis Medical Center
Southeast Missouri Hospital
Columbia
Ellis Fischel State Cancer Hospital
Fort Leonard Wood
U.S. General Leonard Wood Army Hospital
Kansas City
Baptist Memorial Hospital
Menorah Medical Center
St. Luke's Hospital
Trinity Lutheran Hospital
Truman Medical Center
Poplar Bluff
Doctors Regional Medical Center
St. Louis
Deaconess Hospital
Incarnate Word Hospital
Jewish Hospital of St. Louis
St. Anthony's Medical Center
St. Louis Children's Hospital
St. Mary's Health Center
Sikeston
Missouri Delta Community Hospital

Montana
Butte
St. James Community Hospital
Mary Swift Memorial Tumor Clinic

Nebraska
Lincoln
Lincoln General Hospital
Veterans Administration Medical Center
Omaha
Archbishop Bergan Mercy Hospital
Bishop Clarkson Memorial Hospital
Immanuel Medical Center
Nebraska Methodist Hospital
Saint Joseph Hospital
University Hospital & Clinics
University of Nebraska

New Hampshire
Exeter
Exeter Hospital
Hanover
Mary Hitchcock Memorial Hospital
Keene
Cheshire Hospital
Manchester
Catholic Medical Center
Elliot Hospital
Portsmouth
Portsmouth Hospital
Rochester
Frisbie Memorial Hospital

New Jersey
Atlantic City
Atlantic City Medical Center

Belleville
Clara Maass Memorial Hospital
Camden
West Jersey Hospital System
Denville
St. Clare's Hospital
East Orange
Veterans Administration Medical Center
Elizabeth
Elizabeth General Hospital and Dispensary
Wuester Clinic
Englewood
Englewood Hospital
Green Brook
Raritan Valley Hospital
Hackensack
Hackensack Hospital
Hackettstown
Hackettstown Community Hospital
Livingston
St. Barnabas Medical Center
Long Branch
Monmouth Medical Center
Montclair
The Mountainside Hospital
Morristown
Morristown Memorial Hospital
Mount Holly
Burlington County Memorial Hospital
Neptune
Jersey Shore Medical Center—Fitkin Hospital
Newark
Newark Beth Israel Medical Center
Newton
Newton Memorial Hospital
Orange
The Hospital Center at Orange
Passaic
Beth Israel Hospital
Paterson
St. Joseph's Hospital and Medical Center
Phillipsburg
Warren Hospital
Plainfield
Muhlenberg Hospital
Princeton
The Medical Center at Princeton
Somerville
The Somerset Medical Center
Trenton
St. Francis Medical Center
Woodbury
Underwood-Memorial Hospital

New Mexico
Albuquerque
Bernalillo County Medical Center
Lovelace Medical Center
St. Joseph Hospital
Veterans Administration Medical Center

New York
Albany
Veterans Administration Medical Center
Amityville
Brunswick Hospital Center
Binghamton
Our Lady of Lourdes Memorial Hospital

Buffalo
Children's Hospital of Buffalo
Deaconess Hospital
Erie County Medical Center
Roswell Park Memorial Institute
Veterans Administration Medical Center
Castle Point
Veterans Administration Medical Center
Cobleskill
Community Hospital of Schoharie County
Cooperstown
Mary Imogene Bassett Hospital
East Meadow
Nassau County Medical Center
Elmira
Arnot-Ogden Memorial Hospital
Glen Cove
Community Hospital at Glen Cove
Johnson City
Charles S. Wilson Memorial Hospital
Kenmore
Kenmore Mercy Hospital
Manhasset
North Shore University Hospital
Mineola
Nassau Hospital
Mount Kisco
Northern Westchester Hospital Center
Mount Vernon
Mount Vernon Hospital
New Hyde Park
Long Island Jewish-Hillside Medical Center
New Rochelle
New Rochelle Hospital Medical Center
New York City
Bronx *(Mailing address: Bronx)*
Bronx-Lebanon Hospital Center
Misericordia Hospital Medical Center
Montefiore Hospital and Medical Center
Veterans Administration Medical Center
Brooklyn *(Mailing address: Brooklyn)*
Brooklyn Hospital
Jewish Hospital & Medical Center of Brooklyn
Long Island College Hospital
Lutheran Medical Center
St. John's Episcopal Hospital
State University of New York, Downstate Medical Center and Kings County Hospital Center
The Brookdale Hospital Medical Center
The Methodist Hospital
Wyckoff Heights Hospital
Manhattan *(Mailing address: New York)*
Bellevue Hospital Center
Beth Israel Medical Center
Cabrini Medical Center—Columbus Hospital Division
Harlem Hospital Center
Manhattan Eye, Ear and Throat Hospital
Memorial Sloan-Kettering Cancer Center

New York City (cont.)
New York Infirmary—Beekman Downtown Hospital
New York University Medical Center University Hospital
St. Clare's Hospital and Health Center
St. Luke's Hospital Center
St. Vincent's Hospital and Medical Center of New York
The New York Hospital
Veterans Administration Medical Center
Queens (*Mailing address: Astoria, Edgemere, Elmhurst, Far Rockaway, Flushing, Forest Hills, Glen Oaks, Hollis, Jackson Heights, Jamaica, Kew Gardens, Little Neck, Long Island City, Queens Village, St. Albans, and Whitestone)*
Booth Memorial Medical Center, *Flushing*
Flushing Hospital and Medical Center, *Flushing*
Jamaica Hospital, *Jamaica*
LaGuardia Hospital, *Forest Hills*
Mary Immaculate Hospital, Division of the Catholic Medical Center of Brooklyn and Queens, *Jamaica*
Queens Hospital Center, *Jamaica*
St. John's Queens Hospital, Division of the Catholic Medical Center of Brooklyn and Queens, *Elmhurst*
Richmond (*Mailing address: Staten Island)*
Doctors' Hospital of Staten Island
St. Vincent's Medical Center of Richmond
Staten Island Hospital
USPHS Hospital

Nyack
Nyack Hospital

Oceanside
South Nassau Communities Hospital

Patchogue
Brookhaven Memorial Hospital Medical Center

Plainview
Central General Hospital

Port Jefferson
Port Jefferson Combined Cancer Program
John T. Mather Memorial Hospital
St. Charles Hospital

Port Jervis
St. Francis Hospital of Port Jervis, *New York*

Poughkeepsie
Vassar Brothers Hospital

Rochester
Highland Hospital of Rochester
Park Ridge Hospital
Rochester General Hospital
Rochester St. Mary's Hospital of the Sisters of Charity
Strong Memorial Hospital of the University of Rochester
The Genesee Hospital

Rockville Centre
Mercy Hospital

Saratoga Springs
Saratoga Hospital

Schenectady
Ellis Hospital
Syracuse
St. Joseph's Hospital Health Center
University Hospital of Upstate Medical Center
Walton
Delaware Valley Hospital

North Carolina
Asheville
Veterans Administration Medical Center
Camp Le Jeune
Naval Regional Medical Center
Chapel Hill
North Carolina Memorial Hospital
Durham
Duke University Medical Center
Veterans Administration Medical Center
Shelby
Cleveland Memorial Hospital
Valdese
Valdese General Hospital
Winston-Salem
North Carolina Baptist Hospital

North Dakota
Fargo
St. John's Hospital
St. Luke's Hospitals—Fargo Clinic
Grand Forks
The United Hospital
Minot
St. Joseph's Hospital
Rugby
Good Samaritan Hospital Association
Williston
Mercy Hospital

Ohio
Akron
Akron City Hospital
Akron General Medical Center
Cincinnati
Children's Hospital Medical Center
Good Samaritan Hospital
Jewish Hospital of Cincinnati
University of Cincinnati Medical Center, Cincinnati General Hospital
Cleveland
Cleveland Clinic Hospital
Deaconess Hospital of Cleveland
Huron Road Hospital
Lutheran Medical Center
St. Alexis Hospital
Columbus
Children's Hospital
Ohio State University Hospitals
The Hawkes Hospital of Mount Carmel
Mount Carmel Medical Center
Mount Carmel East Hospital
Dayton
Good Samaritan Hospital and Health Center
Miami Valley Hospital
St. Elizabeth Medical Center
Veterans Administration Medical Center
Dover
Union Hospital Association
Kettering
Kettering Memorial Hospital of Kettering Medical Center

Mayfield Heights
Hillcrest Hospital
Sandusky
Good Samaritan Hospital
Springfield
Springfield-Urbana Cancer Program
Community Hospital/Springfield and Clark County
Mercy Medical Center
Mercy Memorial Hospital, *Urbana*
Sylvania
Flower Hospital
Toledo
Medical College of Ohio Hospital
Toledo Hospital
Wright-Patterson AFB
USAF Medical Center
Youngstown
Youngstown Hospital Association

Oklahoma
Ada
Valley View Hospital
Ardmore
Memorial Hospital of Southern Oklahoma
Bartlesville
Jane Phillips Episcopal-Memorial Medical Center
Chickasha
Grady Memorial Hospital
Oklahoma City
Baptist Medical Center of Oklahoma
Mercy Health Center
Oklahoma Children's Memorial Hospital
Presbyterian Hospital
St. Anthony Hospital
South Community Hospital
University Hospitals & Clinics
Okmulgee
Okmulgee Memorial Hospital Authority
Shattuck
Newman Memorial Hospital
Shawnee
Shawnee Medical Center Hospital
Tulsa
Hillcrest Medical Center
Saint Francis Hospital
St. John Medical Center

Oregon
Albany
Albany General Hospital
Bend
St. Charles Medical Center
Coos Bay
Bay Area District Hospital
Corvallis
Good Samaritan Hospital
Eugene
Sacred Heart General Hospital
Grants Pass
Josphine Memorial Hospital
Medford
Medford Tumor Clinic Cancer Program
Providence Hospital
Rogue Valley Memorial Hospital
Oregon City
Willamette Falls Community Hospital
Pendleton
St. Anthony Hospital

Portland
Bess Kaiser Medical Center
Emanuel Hospital
Good Samaritan Hospital and Medical Center
Physicians and Surgeons Hospital
Portland Adventist Medical Center
Providence Medical Center
St. Vincent Hospital and Medical Center
University of Oregon Health Sciences Center Hospital & Clinics
Veterans Administration Medical Center

Salem
Salem Hospital

Tualatin
Meridian Park Hospital

Pennsylvania

Allentown
Allentown and Sacred Heart Hospital Center
Allentown Hospital Association
Sacred Heart Hospital

Altoona
Altoona Hospital
Mercy Hospital

Bethlehem
St. Luke's Hospital

Bryn Mawr
Bryn Mawr Hospital

Danville
Geisinger Medical Center

Drexel Hill
Delaware County Memorial Hospital

Easton
Easton Hospital

Erie
Hamot Medical Center

Franklin
Franklin Hospital

Greensburg
Westmoreland Hospital Association

Johnstown
Conemaugh Valley Memorial Hospital

Lancaster
Lancaster General Hospital
St. Joseph Hospital

Latrobe
Latrobe Area Hospital

Lewistown
Lewistown Hospital

McKeesport
McKeesport Hospital

Natrona Heights
Allegheny Valley Hospital

New Castle
Jameson Memorial Hospital

Norristown
Montgomery Hospital
Sacred Heart Hospital

Paoli
Paoli Memorial Hospital

Philadelphia
Albert Einstein Medical Center—Northern Division
American Oncologic Hospital
Children's Hospital of Philadelphia
Episcopal Hospital
Graduate Hospital
Hahnemann Medical College and Hospital

Philadelphia (*cont.*)
Hospital of the University of Pennsylvania
Jeanes Hospital
Lankenau Hospital
Medical College of Pennsylvania and Hospital
Mercy Catholic Medical Center
Naval Regional Medical Center
Temple University Hospital
Thomas Jefferson University Hospital

Pittsburgh
Allegheny General Hospital
Children's Hospital of Pittsburgh
Magee-Womens Hospital
Mercy Hospital of Pittsburgh
St. Francis General Hospital
St. Margaret Memorial Hospital

Pottsville
Pottsville Hospital and Warne Clinic

Quakertown
Quakertown Community Hospital

Reading
The Reading Hospital and Medical Center

Sayre
Robert Packer Hospital

Scranton
Mercy Hospital

Sellersville
Grand View Hospital

State College
Centre Community Hospital

West Chester
Chester County Hospital

Wilkes-Barre
Veterans Administration Medical Center

York
York Hospital

Rhode Island

Newport
Naval Regional Medical Center

South Carolina

Anderson
Anderson Memorial Hospital

Beaufort
Naval Hospital

Charleston
Medical University of South Carolina

Columbia
Baptist Medical Center at Columbia
Richland Memorial Hospital
Veterans Administration Medical Center

Florence
McLeod Regional Medical Center

Fort Jackson
Moncrief Army Hospital

Greenwood
Self Memorial Hospital

Spartanburg
Spartanburg General Hospital

South Dakota

Aberdeen
St. Luke's Hospital

Watertown
Memorial Medical Center

Yankton
Sacred Heart Hospital

Tennessee

Bristol
Bristol Memorial Hospital
Johnson City
Johnson City Medical Center Hospital, *Mountain Home*
Veterans Administration Medical Center
Knoxville
University of Tennessee Memorial Research Center and Hospital
Memphis
Baptist Memorial Hospital
Methodist Hospitals of Memphis
St. Jude Children's Research Hospital
University of Tennessee/City of Memphis Hospitals
Millington
Naval Regional Medical Center—Memphis
Nashville
George W. Hubbard Hospital and Health Services of Meharry Medical College
Metropolitan Nashville General Hospital
Vanderbilt University Hospital

Texas

Amarillo
Panhandle Regional Tumor Clinic and Registry
High Plains Baptist Hospital
Northwest Texas Hospital
St. Anthony's Hospital
Deaf Smith General Hospital, *Hereford*
Big Spring
Malone-Hogan Hospital
Veterans Administration Medical Center
Corpus Christi
Memorial Medical Center
Naval Regional Medical Center
Spohn Hospital
Dallas
Baylor University Medical Center
Methodist Hospitals of Dallas
Parkland Memorial Hospital—Dallas County Hospital District
St. Paul Hospital
Veterans Administration Medical Center
El Paso
R. E. Thomason General Hospital
William Beaumont Army Medical Center
Fort Sam Houston
Brooke Army Medical Center
Fort Worth
John Peter Smith Hospital
St. Joseph Hospital
Galveston
University of Texas Medical Branch Hospitals
Houston
Ben Taub General Hospital
Park Plaza Hospital
Rosewood General Hospital
St. Elizabeth Hospital
St. Joseph Hospital
Texas Children's Hospital
The University of Texas System Cancer Center, M. D. Anderson Hospital and Tumor Institute

Kerrville
Veterans Administration Medical Center
Lubbock
Highland Hospital
Methodist Hospital
Plainview
Central Plains Regional Hospital
San Antonio
Bexar County Hospital District
Santa Rosa Medical Center
Stephenville
Stephenville Hospital
Temple
King's Daughters Hospital
Scott and White Memorial Hospital
Olin E. Teague Veterans' Center
Waco
Hillcrest Baptist Hospital
Providence Hospital
Wharton
Gulf Coast Medical Center

Utah
Ogden
St. Benedict's Hospital
Salt Lake City
LDS Hospital
University of Utah Medical Center
Veterans Administration Medical Center

Vermont
Burlington
Medical Center Hospital of Vermont
Randolph
Gifford Memorial Hospital

Virginia
Arlington
The Arlington Hospital
Big Stone Gap
Lonesome Pine Hospital
Charlottesville
University of Virginia Hospitals
Danville
The Memorial Hospital
Falls Church
Fairfax Hospital
Hampton
Veterans Administration Medical Center
Harrisonburg
Rockingham Memorial Hospital
Leesburg
Loudoun Memorial Hospital
Low Moor
Alleghany Regional Hospital
Lynchburg
Lynchburg General-Marshall Lodge Hospitals
Virginia Baptist Hospital
Norfolk
DePaul Hospital
Norfolk General Hospital
Portsmouth
Naval Regional Medical Center
Richmond
Medical College of Virginia Hospitals
Virginia Commonwealth University
St. Luke's Hospital
St. Mary's Hospital
Roanoke
Community Hospital of Roanoke Valley

Roanoke Memorial Hospitals

Salem

Lewis-Gale Hospital

Veterans Administration Medical Center

Winchester

Winchester Memorial Hospital

Washington

Aberdeen

Aberdeen Cancer Program

Grays Harbor Community Hospital

St. Joseph Hospital

Bellevue

Overlake Hospital

Bellingham

St. Joseph Hospital

St. Luke's General Hospital

Bremerton

Naval Regional Medical Center

Everett

General Hospital of Everett and Providence Hospital

Kirkland

Evergreen General Hospital

Mount Vernon

Skagit Valley Hospital

Olympia

St. Peter Hospital

Seattle

Children's Orthopedic Hospital & Medical Center

Doctors Hospital

Group Health Cooperative of Puget Sound

Northwest Hospital

Providence Medical Center

Swedish Hospital Medical Center

University Hospital

Virginia Mason Hospital

Sedro Woolley

United General Hospital

Spokane

Deaconess Hospital

Sacred Heart Medical Center

Tacoma

Madigan Army Medical Center

Tacoma General Hospital

Walla Walla

St. Mary Community Hospital

Wenatchee

Wenatchee Valley Clinic

West Virginia

Beckley

Appalachian Regional Hospital

Charleston

Charleston Area Medical Center

Clarksburg

Veterans Administration Medical Center

Elkins

Davis Memorial Hospital

Memorial General Hospital Association

Huntington

St. Mary's Hospital

Veterans Administration Medical Center

Kingwood

Preston Memorial Hospital

Man

Man Appalachian Regional Hospital

Montgomery

Montgomery General Hospital

Morgantown
West Virginia University Hospital
Philippi
Broaddus Hospital
Wheeling
Ohio Valley Medical Center

Wisconsin
Appleton
St. Elizabeth Hospital
Cudahy
Trinity Memorial Hospital
Eau Claire
Luther Hospital
Sacred Heart Hospital
Fond du Lac
St. Agnes Hospital
Green Bay
St. Vincent Hospital
Janesville
Mercy Hospital of Janesville
La Crosse
La Crosse Lutheran Hospital
St. Francis Medical Center
Madison
Madison General Hospital
Methodist Hospital
St. Marys Hospital Medical Center
University of Wisconsin Hospital and Clinics
Manitowoc
Holy Family Hospital
Marinette
Marinette-Menomineé, MI Cancer Program
Marinette General Hospital
Marshfield
Marshfield Clinic
Milwaukee
Columbia Hospital
Deaconess Hospital
Milwaukee County Medical Complex
Mount Sinai Medical Center
St. Francis Hospital
St. Joseph's Hospital
St. Luke's Hospital
St. Mary's Hospital
Monroe
St. Clare Hospital of Monroe
Oshkosh
Mercy Medical Center
Watertown
Watertown Memorial Hospital
Wausau
Wausau Hospital Center
Wood
Veterans Administration Medical Center

Wyoming
Cheyenne
De Paul Hospital
Memorial Hospital of Laramie County

Puerto Rico
Ponce
Clinica Oncologica Andres Grilasca
Hospital De Damas
San German
Hospital De La Concepcion
San Juan
I. Gonzales Martinez Oncologic Hospital
University District Hospital
Veterans Administration Medical Center & Hospital

Appendix C

SUPPORT GROUPS AND INFORMATIONAL ORGANIZATIONS

American Cancer Society, Inc.
777 Third Avenue
New York, NY 10017
212-361-2899

The ACS is an informational organization that also conducts support groups in many areas, which are listed in this section.

Ask a Friend to Explain Reconstruction (AFTER)
1378 Third Avenue
New York, NY 10021
212-472-0040

This group is dedicated to helping women learn about reconstructive breast surgery.

Cancer Consultation Service
237 Thompson Street
New York, NY 10012
212-254-5031

Staffed by members of the Center for Medical Consumers and Judson Memorial Church, this group is offering public access to information about health and healing for cancer patients, their friends and families. There is a reading library, call-in library, counseling and referral services.

CanSurmount

Run by the American Cancer Society, this is a therapeutic program staffed by volunteers. It holds discussion groups, seminars, and guidance in listening.

DES Action
Long Island Jewish Hillside Memorial Center
New Hyde Park, NY 10040
212-343-2222

This self-help group provides information and support for those with DES-related problems, and there are a number of them in the US.

ENCORE—YWCA

A discussion and planned exercise group for postoperative breast cancer patients, held at local units.

HOSPICE
National Hospice Organization
765 Prospect Street
New Haven, Conn 06511

The national hospice may be contacted for names of institutions where hospice programs exist in the United States.

I Can Cope

This is a group of the American Cancer Society aimed at meeting the educational and psychological needs of people with cancer.

Make Today Count
P.O. Box 303
Burlington, Iowa 52601
319-735-6112

The goal of this group is to help cancer patients and their families "live each day as fully and completely as possible." To do so it is an organization of self-help to meet emotional needs.

NATIONAL CANCER INSTITUTE
National Cancer Institute
Office of Cancer Communications
Bethesda, Maryland 21205
800-638-6694

For current information on study groups, nutritional support, and emotional support groups, you may contact NCI at any time.

National Women's Health Network
224 Seventh Street, S.E.
Washington, D.C. 20003

An organization concerned with the rights of women in terms of health care and in understanding cancer. It is a national consumer group devoted exclusively to women and their health needs.

Reach to Recovery

This is a volunteer group of women who have undergone mastectomies, and who devote their time to helping women in hospitals and at home adjust to the trauma of breast surgery. It is a program of the American Cancer Society.

Women's Breast Cancer Advisory Center
11426 Rockville Pike
Suite 406
Rockville, MD 20850

Founded and run by Rose Kushner, author of *Why Me?*, the center is a non-profit, consumer-oriented organization that provides information on all aspects of breast diseases—especially cancer.

Appendix D

The chart below gives an overview of the detection of and outlook for the cancers that most often affect women.

Good News in Detection—Treatment	*High-Risk Groups*	*Warning and Safeguard*
BREAST—Most tumors detectable through the breast self-examination. Newer tests include graphic stress telethermography and now reduced radiation exposure with mammography.	• Lump or nipple discharge. • History of breast cancer in family. • Over age 35; especially over 50. • Never had children; first child after age 30.	• Lump or thickening in the breast, or unusual discharge from nipple. —Regular checkup, monthly breast self-exam.
ENDOMETRIAL—Newer screening methods and office biopsy techniques. These include: Endometrial aspiration biopsy, biopsy, Gravlee jet washer, the Vabra aspiration, and other similar techniques.	• Late menopause (after age 55). • Diabetes, high blood pressure and overweight. • Age 50+.	• Unusual bleeding or discharge. —Regular check-up, including pelvic examination with PAP test and endometrial biopsy.
CERVIX—Nearly 100% cure rate during the preinvasive stage. New techniques allow for minimal surgery: the cone biopsy, freezing technique, electro-caudery and local surgery with laser.	• Frequent sex in early teens or with many partners. • Low socio-economic background. • Genital herpes.	• Unusual bleeding or discharge. —Regular check-up, PAP test.
OVARIAN—Response rate 70% in what was once thought to be incurable achieved through new drug combinations such as cis-platinum and adriamycin.	• History of ovarian cancer among close relatives. • Aged 50+. • Never had children.	• Vague symptoms of gastric disorders. —Regular check-ups.

VULVA—Greater awareness by physicians and patients with earlier detection.	• Women over 60. • Possibly women with early menopause. • Genital herpes.	• Any sore, ulcer or raised lesion which does not respond to local treatment within two weeks. —Regular check-ups.
VAGINA—Application of reconstruction techniques continues to improve.	• DES-exposed women. • Post-menopausal women.	• Unusual bleeding. —Prompt check-up if symptom occurs.
OTHER CANCERS AFFECTING WOMEN		
COLON—RECTUM—A self-testing kit being used in experiments on high-risk persons. Cure rate 70% when treated during earliest stage. For some patients, spinchter-saving muscle surgery available in later stages.	• History of rectal polyps. • Rectal polyps run in family. • History of ulcerative colitis. • Blood in stool. • Over age 40.	• Change in bowel habits; bleeding. —Regular check-up, including digital, ococult blood and proctoscopic exams, especially after age 40.
LUNG—Fiberoptic bronchoscope available for some cases. Combination chemotherapy for oat cell has remarkable remission rate when detected early. Best news for common forms of lung cancer—Anti-Smoking Campaigns.	• Heavy cigarette smoker over age 50. • Started cigarette smoking age 15 or before. • Smoker working with or near asbestos.	• Persistent cough or lingering respiratory ailment. —80% of lung cancer would be prevented if no one smoked cigarettes.

Chart and figures derived from American Cancer Society 1981. Reference Chart and information from JAMA and *New England Journal of Medicine*

Postscript

We have tried to keep the material in this book current and accurate, but it is impossible for the printed word to be completely up-to-date in an area as dynamic as that covered in this book. Achievements in basic science and advances in clinical applications are made rapidly and tomorrow's newspapers may report major breakthroughs. But do not be lured away from sound, competent medical advice by the promise of a new and unproven "cure," and do not accept "miracle" cures offered by those who are over-critical of the medical establishment that has produced so much progress. Hopefully, many of the areas of difficulty mentioned in this book will yield to medical investigations, and we look forward to the continued progress of the art and science of medicine in the care of malignancy in women.

RCW

Index